THE
BODYSENSE DIET

THE
BODYSENSE DIET

*Tune into your body's own power
and lose weight naturally*

Judith Wills

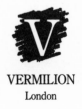

VERMILION
London

1 3 5 7 9 10 8 6 4 2

Text copyright © Judith Wills 1997
Photographs copyright © Random House UK Ltd 1997

First published in the United Kingdom in 1997 by Vermilion
an imprint of Ebury Press
Random House
20 Vauxhall Bridge Road
London SW1V 2SA

Random House Australia (Pty) Limited
20 Alfred Street, Milsons Point, Sydney,
New South Wales 2061, Australia

Random House New Zealand Limited
18 Poland Road, Glenfield
Auckland 10, New Zealand

Random House South Africa (Pty) Ltd
Endulini, 5a Jubilee Road,
Parktown 2193, South Africa

Random House UK Limited Reg. No. 954009

A CIP catalogue record for this book is available from the British Library

ISBN: 0 09 181459 6

Printed and bound in Great Britain by
Cox & Wyman Ltd, Reading, Berkshire

CONTENTS

INTRODUCTION

These days you rarely hear the word 'sensible' mentioned in the same breath as the word 'diet'. Dieting for women is more usually thought of as *not* sensible – more likely to do harm than good.

That view is often partially justified. There have been a lot of bad and silly diets offered over the decades; there have been very many women whose lives and self-confidence have probably been made worse by dieting, not better.

But, at a time when the number of seriously overweight women is increasing rapidly, rather than to say, simply don't diet, the answer is to provide a system for women that *is* sensible. Safe. Practical. Easy to follow. Enjoyable, even! *A plan to accommodate the way women's bodies really are.*

I talked to many women to confirm their feelings about food and dieting; their worries about their bodies; their beliefs about exercise; their problems and their misconceptions about slimming. And, having listened, I wrote *Bodysense.*

I have subtitled it *The Ultimate Diet for Women* because I do believe that is what it is. It shows you how to tune into your body's own signals and use what you learn to give your body what it needs at any given time. When the conflict that accompanies most dieting is taken away, you will lose weight *quite naturally.*

With *Bodysense*, you will learn to plug into your body's own power and use it, not fight it.

With *Bodysense* you will learn to be *kind* to your body both while you slim and afterwards, in keeping the weight off.

You will also learn not to expect too much of yourself; to set goals that really are achievable.

Listen to your body.
Learn to feel proud of it.
And find your true shape – quite naturally.

1

TAKE A FRESH LOOK AT YOUR BODY

So you want to be in good shape? But what, exactly, *is* 'good shape' . . . for *you*?

The first aim of *Bodysense* is to help you to know what you are likely to achieve with your own body, and to teach you not to expect miracles. For it is a sad fact that few women are realistic about their own bodies.

Listen to these women talking:

'Before I was 25 I used always to be 57kg (8 stone 12lbs). But since then I've put on nearly 6.4kg (a stone) and I spend my whole life trying to get back to 8 stone 12, which I know is my right weight. That's when I looked my best.'
– *Anne*, 35.

'I have inherited my mother's big pear shape – my waist is only 60cm (24in) but my hips are 97.5cm (39in) and I will try anything going – creams, massage, machines, exercise, to get them down to my ideal of 90cm (36in). Something's going to work eventually.'
– *Maria*, 25.

'I weigh 54kg (8$^{1}/_{2}$ stone) and I'm 1.64m (5ft 4ins). Everyone else says I look fine, but when I look in the mirror I see bumps and bulges. I keep seeing clothes in the shops that would look better on me if I were 51kg (8 stone).'
– *Pamela*, 29.

These three women, each acquaintances of mine, do not, in reality, have a weight or shape problem – except in their own minds.

The first step towards acquiring a shape and size you can keep for ever is to be realistic. Stop defying your body's natural status; stop fighting for it to be something it can't, naturally or happily, be.

· *You and Your Natural Weight* ·

So first, let's look at your approximate natural body weight.

Although much has been written about the folly of aiming to be too thin (and feminists have made slimness virtually Politically Incorrect), many women do still consider thinness as an ideal. Straight away, let me tell you that it is *not*.

Never mind the 'correctness' or otherwise of it – there are far more sensible reasons for not aiming to be thin.

Your health

Contrary to what you may believe, it is not necessarily healthy to be thin. In fact, extreme thinness is as unhealthy – and predisposes you to as many illnesses and problems – as extreme fatness. For example, extreme thinness can promote earlier menopause and more menopausal symptoms, can cause irregular periods or cessation of periods, and can increase your risk of osteoporosis in later life. This latter is not only because thin women's bodies don't contain as much bone mass as fatter women's do, but also because thin women have less natural oestrogen (the female hormone), which is the body's own protection against calcium loss.

Thin people are also more at risk from infectious diseases. And, of course, if you stay thin by eating like a sparrow, you may well suffer from various nutritional deficiencies which may lead to health problems.

It is hard for women to get enough of all the nutrients we need in our diet unless we eat a reasonable amount of food – and many women stay thin on far less than a 'reasonable amount'.

For instance, it is not easy for a woman to get her daily recommended intake of iron (13mg a day) even on a normal diet of around 1,950 calories. Reduce that to 800 or 1,000, as many women do, cut out red meat, as many women do, and unless you make a determined, well-informed effort, you will almost certainly fall short of iron and may end up with anaemia; especially if you have heavy periods.

That is just one example – there are many more, and we'll be looking at your diet in detail later in the book.

You can even – and this will shock all of you who have religiously tried to eliminate all fat from your diet for years – be deficient in *fat*. Fat is an important source of the fat-soluble vitamins A, D and E, and your body needs a certain amount of fat to help these vitamins to be absorbed. Your body also needs essential fatty acids – special fats found in certain plant foods and fishes.

The World Health Organisation sets a lowest fat intake for women at 15% of total energy intake – that's about 32g (1oz) of fat a day for a woman on an average calorie level.

I should say a word here about women who stay thin while eating plenty. This isn't all that common. People who stay thin and seem to eat a lot, often don't, in fact, eat as much as they seem to, because they tend to fill up on the lower-calorie foods, or take smaller portions. However, it is true that some women *are* naturally thin. These women either have a very high metabolic rate, or burn a lot of calories through activity, and my comments on health and thinness may not apply to them.

But the fact is that, for most women, once we head into our late twenties, thirties, forties and beyond, it is not wise to attempt to maintain a thin frame, especially if it means existing on a meagre diet.

Your well-being

I know one or two women who are beanpole slim and look terrific in whatever they wear. They are smart, well groomed and have maintained a size 10 or lower for many years.

But do I envy them? No, I don't. Because I know exactly how little pleasure they get from their meals to maintain that weight; how terrified they are if the scales register so much as a 450g (1lb) weight gain; how, every time someone says to them, 'How lovely it must be not to have to watch your weight,' they feel like screaming because, in reality, they watch their weight every waking minute of every day. And, as the years go by, they have to eat less and less to maintain that weight.

That's not enjoyment of life; that's not something to aim for – that's more like a prison sentence.

I also know several women who are always dieting but never quite manage to lose the last few pounds to get down to what they consider their 'right' weight – like Anne and Pamela. Or they get there for a few days or weeks but never maintain it for long.

That's because *they are already at their right weight. Their bodies aren't meant to be thin.*

So for all these women – millions of women – thinness, if they have it, means pleasure at a very big price, and if they don't have it, it means years of dissatisfaction – with themselves, their bodies – and their lives. What a waste of time!

This chapter will help you to discover just how slim you were meant to be. Once you've discovered that, don't even think of trying to get your weight down below what is right for you.

Keep telling yourself (start now): 'I do not want to be thin.'

And, when that is firmly fixed in your mind, we can go on ...

In case by now you are wondering whether this really is a 'diet' book or not – let me reassure you. I don't want you to be fat, either.

Just as you have a natural weight below which it is unwise to be, so you have an approximate weight and size above which there is no need to be – for your health, your happiness, or whatever. I do not believe that to be fat is to be happy. I know that humans were not made to be huge, or flabby, or slothful.

While there is no harm at all in going up a dress size – or a stone – in between your slim youth and your middle age, too much weight gain brings so many health problems, that to be fat when you needn't be is plainly masochistic.

Indeed, the latest research indicates that being as little as 11kg (22lb) over your 18-year-old weight may start to produce increased risk of heart disease. And at 20kg (40lb) over your 18-year-old weight, health risks increase sevenfold.

Health problems linked with fatness are: heart disease and strokes, arthritis, mid-life onset of diabetes, high blood pressure, muscular pains, varicose veins, shortness of breath, infertility, immobility, gallstones and some forms of cancer. For women, breast, ovarian and uterine cancer are more common in the obese.

If you are fat and 20, these problems may not be apparent, but as the years go by, the risks increase – especially as most people who are overweight when young tend to continue putting on more and more as they get older. In other words, a two-stone weight problem at 20 will probably be a six-stone weight problem at 40.

Women naturally have more body fat than men: 18–25% is average compared with 10–15% for men. Women are naturally curvier than men, with narrower waists, wider hips and more fat around the upper arms, bottom and thighs (and, of course, the breasts).

That is why it is silly for most women to hanker after the 'straight up and down' look. And because you are curvy, that doesn't mean you can't also be well toned, firm-muscled and fit.

What we want to achieve is nothing more than a reasonable, realistic balance for *you*. A weight that is within the bounds of 'average' or 'normal' – which gives enough leeway to stop anyone having to worry about half a stone or so. We want you to feel happy – with a weight you can easily maintain *naturally*. So now let's find out . . .

Are you overweight?

There are various ways to find the answer to this. Surprisingly enough, the bathroom scales – especially if you are, or think you are, only slightly fat – are not necessarily the best indicator; or, at least, not on their own. The height/weight charts that everyone has used since the Sixties are rather out of date now.

Instead, I want you to follow the steps below until you get to the point at which you can reach a firm conclusion.

· *Step One* ·

Work out your Body Mass Index

Your Body Mass Index (BMI) is the index most professionals will use to determine whether or not you are overweight. And, used with a certain amount of common sense, it is a good indicator.

To work out your own BMI, you divide your weight in kilograms by your height in metres squared.

(Convert weight in pounds into kilograms by dividing by 2.2. Convert height into metres by multiplying your inch height by 0.025. To square your height, it is easiest to use a calculator.)

Example: You weigh 66kg (10 stone 5lbs). You are 1.72 metres (5ft 7ins) tall. Squared, this is 2.8. Your BMI is $66 \div 2.8$, which works out at 23.5 (to the nearest 0.5).

This is the international classification of BMIs:

Below 20: Underweight.

   20–25: Acceptable weight range.

   25–30: Overweight.

   30–40: Obese.

Over 40: Very obese.

If your BMI is over 30, I can tell you straight away that you should lose some weight. You can move straight on to the 'You and Your Natural Shape' section on page 19 of this chapter, then follow the *Bodysense* plan in the rest of the book.

If your BMI is under 20, then you don't need to lose any weight. If it is, and you *think* you do, then I would suggest that you get in touch with your GP who, depending upon where you live, can put you in touch with a therapist or class specialising in body image problems.

Between 20 and 30, the picture isn't quite so clear which is why your result needs sensible interpretation.

For most women, a BMI of between 20 and 25 means that you do not need to lose any weight, certainly not for your health and probably not for your looks. If you think you do, it could be that your body is in need of toning up – what looks like flab may just be poor muscle tone, in which case, turn to the 'You and Your Natural Shape' section on page 19.

But for some women, it is possible to have a BMI of under 25 and a requirement, for the sake of your health, to lose a little weight. This is if you take the next test and find that you have a large Waist to Hip Ratio (WHR), which will mean that you are carrying a disproportionately large amount of fat around your middle, with slim hips and/or thin limbs. So BMIs of between 20 and 25 should do the WHR test that follows just as an extra check.

If your WHR result is low and your BMI 25 or under, think no more about losing weight. You may want to tone up, but you don't want to slim. Okay?

That leaves all of you whose BMI is between 25 and 30 – and, I suspect, that is the majority of you. This is the area that needs the most careful interpretation of all.

The closer to 25 your BMI, the least likely it is that you need to lose some weight for the sake of your health. The nearer to 30 your BMI is, the more likely it is that you do need to lose weight.

All of you in the 25 to 30 BMI bracket need to do the WHR test that follows and use it in conjunction with your BMI result to determine whether you need to be slimmer, because weight distribution, particularly if you are not very overweight, is as important as the weight itself.

So, let's move on to the Waist to Hip Ratio (WHR) test now.

· *Step Two* ·

Take the Waist to Hip Ratio test

An excellent measure of the likely health risk of your surplus weight, is the Waist to Hip Ratio. This measures the distribution of your fat.

Body fat that lies around your waist and stomach is much more closely linked to heart disease and other health problems than fat that is carried on other parts of the body. Pear-shaped women with big hips and thighs but relatively small waists are, for example, much less at risk than the pot-bellied person with relatively slim hips and legs.

The hour-glass figure, with a good covering of fat on the shoulders, bust, bottom and legs but with a trim waist is a healthy female look.

The hour-glass woman may weigh the same as, or more than, a woman who has little surplus body fat on her – except round her middle. The hour-glass woman will have a low WHR, the fat-bellied woman, a high WHR. And the latter may be storing up trouble for herself, along with that fat around her middle. And that is why, if your BMI does not conclusively prove that you are too fat or too thin, the WHR test is an important one.

To find out your WHR, all you do is measure your waist around its smallest point and your hips around their largest point, and then divide your waist measurement in inches or centimetres, by your hip measurement in inches or centimetres (but don't mix imperial and metric measurements).

Examples:

Your waist is 77.5cm (31ins) and your hips are 100cm (40ins). Your WHR is 0.77.

Your waist is 70cm (28ins) and your hips 85cm (34ins). Your WHR is 0.82.

Your waist is 77.5cm (31ins) and your hips 95cm (38ins). Your WHR is 0.81.

An 'average' WHR for women is 0.80. Below that means that you have a low WHR, above that means that you have a high WHR – and the closer your WHR gets to 1.0, the bigger your waist is in relation to your hips, and the more at risk you are of ill health, particularly coronary disease. And the more likely it is that you are overweight and unfit.

Now let's look at your WHR in conjunction with your BMI ascertained in Step One.

- If your BMI was 25 or under but your WHR is high, you are probably a natural 'skinny' (Ectomorph – see page 20) who has over the years thickened around the middle while keeping your slim arms and legs. No matter what the scales tell you, you do need to do something about that tum – you are an 'apple-shape', albeit not a fat apple, and apple shape is risk shape. The interesting thing is that the Waist to Hip Ratio used to be considered a 'male' test – for it was classically men who suffered from the 'pot belly' syndrome, with small chest, weedy legs but a big, fat middle. Now more women are becoming apple-shaped and more prone to the same health problems as men. For instance, heart disease is on the increase among women of all ages.
- If your BMI is between 25 and 30 and your WHR is high, you are also more prone to health problems than a mildly overweight person of pear-shape, so it is important to lose

weight from around your middle and take some exercise. If you don't, your waist will just go on getting bigger and bigger as you get older.

● If your BMI is between 25 and 30 and your WHR is low, you may have a 'hip and thigh' weight problem. You are a natural pear-shape and your surplus weight poses much less of a health risk for you than if it were around your middle. Read the section headed 'You and your natural shape' and carry on and answer the questions in the rest of this section to see if you ought to slim. As a rule of thumb, the nearer your BMI is to 30, even if your WHR is low, the more likely it is that you could do with losing some weight.

· *Step Three* ·

Common-sense questions

If I have advised you to carry on through this section – or if you're still not sure whether you are overweight, ask yourself the following questions and record the answers.

1 *How old are you?*
Assuming you are an adult (this book isn't intended for children and young teenagers), it is acceptable to gain a stone or so over the years between young adulthood and late middle age (if, of course, you weren't fat as a young adult). So if, for instance, you were 58kg (9 stone) and 1.62m (5ft 3ins) tall at 25 (giving you a BMI of 23) and are now 55 and 64kg (10 stone), with a BMI of 25.5, that is a reasonable weight for your *age*, especially if the weight has come on slowly and you still exercise.

However, if you are 1.62m (5ft 3ins) tall, and weighed 58kg (9 stone) aged 20 with a BMI of 23, and are now 30 and weigh 70kg (11 stone), with a BMI of just over 28, you have gained quite a lot of weight in a relatively short space of time, and the likelihood is that if you don't do something about it now, by 40 you will have put on another 12.8kg (2 stone) and have a BMI of over 33.

In other words, try to relate your current weight to your current age and to what you used to weigh as a young adult.

2 *What size are your blood relatives?*

Although different members of the same family can be different
sizes and shapes, looking at your parents and your brothers and
sisters can be a good guide as to whether your natural weight is
slimmer than you currently are. Are they all, or mostly, of slim
build? Or are they all large-framed and well-covered? This isn't a
foolproof question, as some all-large families are simply all over-
fed and/or take too little exercise. But, if the family are all slim,
and you are the only large one, it is quite likely that your genetic
predisposition is not to be large but to be slim. An honest
appraisal of your eating habits compared with other members of
your family will in that case confirm or deny the concept.

3 *Do you feel fit and healthy?*

If you feel generally well, take plenty of exercise and know you are
fit, with an average or low WHR, a BMI over 25 is probably
nothing to worry about.

However, if you feel sluggish, breathless, and generally out of
sorts, more exercise and a healthier diet may be at least part of the
answer.

4 *Do you eat well?*

Sounds an obvious question, but if you already eat a healthy diet,
with plenty of fresh fruit and vegetables, lean protein, fibre, and
not too much saturated fat or junk foods, and have a BMI of
between 25 and 30, you may have a naturally larger build than
other women.

Now look at your answers to the four questions together. If you
are, say, 50, with large relatives, you feel fit and healthy, you take
regular exercise and you eat a healthy diet, your BMI of between
25 and 30 may be fine, especially if your WHR is low or average,
and especially if your BMI is nearer 25 than 30.

However, if you are, say, 30, with slim relatives, you don't feel
particularly fit and well, you take little exercise, you know you eat
far too many chocolates (or whatever!) and you have a high WHR
– and especially if your BMI is nearer 30 than 25 – then the
likelihood is that you should lose at least a little weight.

Be honest with yourself – it's your body, after all.

· *You and Your Natural Shape* ·

We've looked at your weight, and I am sure that you now know whether you need to lose weight or not. Sometimes it is hard to separate your weight and your size from your shape.

In fact, more women seem to worry about their body shape than they do about its size. You know the scenario – even if you haven't a kilogram of spare flesh on you, you will despair of your short legs, or your thick ankles, or your short waist, or your small bust. . . etc., etc. Every one of us, it seems, dislikes something about our body shape.

I did it myself, for years. I hated my 67.5cm (27ins) waist for not being 60cm (24ins), and I hated my over-skinny calves (as I saw it). Not thanking my mother for my reasonable bust, or my father for my long legs, I just moaned about the imperfections, wanting to look like what appeared to be perfect models in the women's magazines.

I want new genes!

Yet if I had spent two minutes considering my mother's shape and my father's shape, I would have seen straight away that tiny waists and ballet-dancers' calves just don't figure in our family genes.

Our basic body shape is decided for us before we are born, by who our parents are, what shape they are, and which characteristics from each parent have been programmed into the fertilised egg that is to become us.

Other factors, such as how good a diet we are fed in the womb and as babies, how much exercise we take as children and how healthy we are also affect our looks.

By the time we have finished growing into adults, there is nothing we can do to alter our basic bone structure, or our height. And there is nothing we can do to alter our genetic predisposition to, say, wide hips, a big bust, short thighs, long fingers or whatever it is that makes us different from the next person.

Yes, I can get my waist as slim as it can be through the right diet and exercise – but because of the way I was made, I am never going to have a 60cm (24ins) waist. So why on earth did I spend years feeling almost guilty that I wasn't able to achieve it? I can – and have – built a small amount of muscle in my calves through the right exercise . . . but they are never going to be dancer's calves whatever I do. It doesn't matter. And, even if it did matter, what would be the point of worrying about something beyond my control?

I suppose today some people *do* achieve the impossible – bodies that aren't naturally feasible for them – through things like cosmetic reduction, implants, liposuction and so on. But where is the satisfaction in acquiring a shape that isn't really yours? Strangely enough, the women most likely to be desperate enough to alter their bodies through unnatural means are the ones who were most nearly perfect in the first place. But no one, absolutely no one in the world *is* perfect.

So the point from which we start in this book is making sure that you know that you can't have a perfect body.

You can have a fit body; a great body; an individual body that is yours and that you can be proud of – but there really is no such thing as perfection. So stop worrying about things you can't change, and let's take a look at what you *can* change.

Your body type

Basic body shape is often categorised into three classic types:

The Ectomorph The ectomorph is the slimmest of the body types, with a tendency to find it hard to build muscle or to put on fat. Limbs are often long, waist is often thick in comparison to bust and hips. Wrists, ankles, fingers and toes may be long and slim; elbows and knees may be bony. Bust may be small, neck long. In later years, weight may come on more easily, especially around the midriff. In sport, the ectomorph shines most in long-distance sports, long jump, high jump, basketball.

The Mesomorph The classic mesomorph is of chunky, muscular build with a high muscle to body fat ratio. Shoulders are square and powerful, the body looks strong, firm, well proportioned. The mesomorph has plenty of energy and strength, often with well-developed legs and buttocks, broad neck and flat stomach. The mesomorph female will probably be good at sprinting, gymnastics, and a good all-rounder in many sports and activities.

The Endomorph The endomorph looks well rounded even when not overweight. The female endomorph has well-covered shoulders, smooth, plump arms and legs without great muscle definition, curvy bust and hips even when slim and often a small waist when young. The endomorph puts on weight quite easily as she gets older, especially as she is not naturally sporty. She prefers non-organised sport such as dancing.

Most of us don't fit neatly into just one of the three categories but are a combination – typically one type dominant with a second type mixed in. Few of us are all three in equal amounts, and for most of us it isn't difficult to spot our predominant type. Once spotted, it is wisest to try to *adapt* to that natural shape and work with it, rather than to try to change yourself completely – it won't work!

For example, if you're predominantly endomorph, you should learn to like your curves, but that isn't to say you shouldn't find some exercise you can enjoy and build a little more muscle definition to help you to keep the pounds at bay by speeding up your natural metabolic rate slightly.

You may not win prizes for your athletic ability but you'll be doing yourself a favour, which is what matters most.

If you are a muscular mesomorph, it's no use hankering after the figure of Elle McPherson, because she is a classic ectomorph with a little endomorph in her. You should simply eat wisely, get plenty of exercise to work off all that energy, and be thankful for the fact that mesomorphs have strong bones, strong muscles and, of the three types, the greatest natural ability to stay fit.

If you are an ectomorph, forget about turning yourself into Sharron Davies (a classic mesomorph), but remember you should do all the strength and tone exercises you can to help build up strong bones and a little muscle. You can eat plenty without putting on weight, at least when you are young (though watch that middle as you grow older).

Rule one. Work with what you've got.

Flab versus fat

If you are endomorphic, you are likely to look 'softer' than a mesomorph or ectomorph, but we can all suffer from body flab because of under-used and out-of-tone muscles, and this can not only give the impression of fatness even if we aren't overweight, but can also alter our natural body shape for the worse.

So it is important to admit it if you have flab. How do you find out?

Well, stand in your underwear or naked in front of a full-length mirror, and let's find out.

- Hold your arms up and out to either side. Have you wobbly flesh under the upper arms when you shake your arms about? Or can you actually see a fold of flesh hanging down off your upper arm? 'Yes' to either of those questions means your upper arms are in bad need of toning and strength work.

- Stand and look at your stomach. Is there any hint of sagginess around the lower abdomen where it meets your hips at either side? Stand sideways and look. Even after tucking your stomach in as far as you can by using any muscle you can locate there, and by tilting your pelvic cage to improve your posture, does your stomach stick out a lot? If so, you can achieve a much better shape to your midriff with the right toning exercises.

- Look at your legs. Keeping your feet still, shake your legs from side to side. Does flesh on your inner thighs wobble? You can tone that up and improve thigh shape considerably with toning work.

- Are your legs pretty shapeless even though not fat? Even ectomorphs can add shape and definition to their legs through aerobic and toning work.

- Does your bottom look flat and saggy? You can make it higher and firmer with the right exercise.

- Stand sideways on to see if your shoulders droop into a letter 'c', making you look fatter than you are. If so, the right exercises will correct your posture.

If you answered 'yes' to any of these questions, your shape and tone can be improved with the exercise programme in Chapter Seven. The improvement may be vast, or not so vast, depending on what the problems are. For instance, a flabby stomach, if worked upon with the right exercises, will always show quicker and more noticeable improvement than flabby thighs. But you *can* improve any shape problem connected to poor muscle tone and/or poor body posture.

In fact, it's worth talking about your posture (or body alignment) in a little more detail as it affects your shape more than you think.

Very few of us carry our bodies in the way they were meant to be carried – we stand incorrectly, sit incorrectly and, over the years, our muscles adapt to the incorrect things we are asking them to do by compensating . . . building extra muscle somewhere to take the extra strain that imbalances have caused; stretching out muscle somewhere else. . . . A simple example is the person who doesn't stand up with a straight spine, but stoops. Over the years, the back of neck muscles will become overdeveloped in order to try to hold the head up (the head should be balanced on the spine, not forcibly held up by muscle) and the muscles surrounding the shoulder blades will become elongated and weak. The chest muscles will also become short and tight.

So our shape is affected by poor body alignment. And almost every part of the body can be affected – chest, neck, shoulders, upper back, lower back, bottom, stomach, thighs, knees, calves, feet. Long-term poor posture causes poor shape.

But the good news is that, however entrenched your poor posture habits are, they can be reversed – although not overnight. By working the under-used muscles and stretching the overworked muscles; by re-aligning yourself consciously as often as you think about it every day, you can put your body back as it was meant to be.

Chapters Six and Seven give you all the help you will need on your shape. In as little as two hours a week you can shape yourself up within the boundaries of your own body.

But remember – your shape is *your* shape. And it's going to take time to improve. *Bodysense*, as I said at the beginning of this chapter, is about being realistic. It's about *us* working with what *you've* got; about *us* achieving the best for *you*.

Other people's bodies are their own business.

Let's look after *you*.

2

Now Tune into Your Body Signals

Why do we spend so much time and effort in fighting our bodies; defying our bodies; ignoring our body signalling to us what it really needs?

Melanie is a 32-year-old who spends her life putting on and taking off half a stone, alternately overfeeding her body on binge carbohydrate foods like biscuits, and starving it on oranges.

'I go on a strict diet four times a year to lose weight – my favourite is just citrus fruit, nothing else – and it always works. Ideally, I'd like to lose a stone, but I never manage to stay on the diet for more than 10 days; after that I binge. I get headaches, too, when I'm dieting – but that's all right, isn't it? It's detox working.'

Says Karen, 29, 'I stick to a good diet and fitness programme for most of the time, but every single month I end up hating myself because I can't do it for the last week or so before my period.

'I weigh myself every day, and as the month goes on I manage to lose less and less weight, however good I am. Then in that week before my period, I put on about 2kg (4lbs) – more than I've lost in the whole month. So next month I have to start all over again. I hate it. I hate myself. Sometimes I wish I were male.'

Melanie and Karen aren't unusual; they are typical women with typical attitudes to their own struggles with their bodies.

They – we all – must learn to read our body signals and be kind to our bodies.

Headaches through dieting aren't wonderful 'detox' symptoms – they are your body's way of telling you that you aren't giving it enough carbohydrate and probably not enough liquid, either.

Fluid retention before a period is a natural phenomenon for

most women, to be handled and minimised with care and knowledge.

Bingeing is not a sign of weakness or failure; it is a sign that your body is crying out for food because it has been undernourished.

The female body is a powerful human factory; converting food into energy, manufacturing hormones; for a large part of your life, getting itself ready to have children; rewarding you if you help it to be strong and healthy; complaining if you mistreat it.

But few of us ever really bother to understand what is going on in our bodies, and even fewer to read the signals of distress or thanks that it puts out.

In this chapter you aim to get your brain and your body on the same wavelength. You want your body to look good and feel good. To achieve that, you need to be *kind* to your body. You need to be realistic; not just about your ideal weight and your best shape, as we learnt in Chapter One, but also about the journey to get there.

Tune into your body and let it *help* you. *Read the signals.* Then, and only then, will you be able to lose weight naturally, and for good.

· *Keep a Body Diary* ·

First I would like you to start keeping a 'body diary', like the one below, every day for the next month. Don't worry, you can start it now, continue reading the book and follow the *Bodysense* plan. But when you have finished the diary you can look back over it and pick out your own natural body patterns and rhythms and this will help you to recognise in yourself the *Bodysense* concept.

It will only take a few minutes a day to fill in, and I think you will enjoy it. It is the start of paying attention to yourself and your body. It will teach you to look out for signals and answer them or adapt to them.

Fill it in at the end of each day. The ideal is to use a 'page to a day' diary. Here's an example:

DATE: Monday 2nd May.

Circumstances: Ordinary working day; very busy as usual.

Body notes: Felt good; full of energy, though rushed.

Mind notes: Mind felt good, too – alert, positive. Nothing seemed to get me down.

Eating notes: Had usual breakfast; sandwich for lunch; ready meal in evening; didn't feel hungry all day. Didn't think about food, really.

Exercise notes: Did nothing at all except rush to and from work. Didn't think about it.

*Cycle notes**: Day 5.

Here's another example of the same woman's diary three weeks later:

DATE: Monday 23rd May.

Circumstances: Ordinary working day, though quite quiet.

Body notes: Felt fat and lethargic. Job to stay awake after lunch.

Mind notes: Felt on a bit of a short fuse and couldn't make decisions. Ended day with a list of tasks I should have done and hadn't, which made me more annoyed still.

Eating notes: Skipped breakfast because I felt fat; ate chocolate bar mid-morning. Felt need for carbs at lunchtime and had a huge croissant filled with honey. Too tired to cook a meal in the evening; had a takeaway. It was horrible.

Exercise notes: Did nothing, of course. Didn't feel up to it.

*Cycle notes**: Day 26.

You will see, as your diary takes shape, that all kinds of factors are at work influencing how well you eat, how many calories you consume, what activity you do. Make your diary as detailed as you can. Here are some notes to help you to fill it in:

Circumstances: Note where you are and what you are doing today, e.g., is it work or leisure time; a typical day or an abnormal day? Were you sedentary or dashing around?

---

* This is for if you have a monthly menstrual cycle. Day 1 is the third day of your period and the days continue in sequence until you begin Day 1 again on the third day of your next period. Depending on the length of your cycle, then, you may have anything from 20-something to 40 or more days in your cycle. The average cycle is 28 days but women vary greatly. If you do not have periods, ignore cycle notes.

Body: Note how you felt physically. Fit? Strong? Lethargic? Weak? Energetic? Poor body image? Good body image? Any aches and pains or tenderness? Rested? Relaxed? Tensed? Weary?

Mind notes: Did you wake up positive or negative? Happy or sad? Frightened or calm? Tired or zestful? How did you cope with crises or surprises?

Eating notes: Give a quick résumé of what you ate, why, and how you felt about it. Was it a healthy eating day? Did you eat different food from what you'd intended? Did you overeat/ undereat? Did you think about food a lot or hardly at all? Did you feel hungry, sated, ravenous? Did you crave a particular food? Did your eating today make you feel good or bad about yourself?

Exercise notes: Did you take any activity today and, if so, what? How did it make you feel? How well did you do? How hard did you try?

Making a graph

By the time you have completed a month or so of your diary, you will see that your body, your eating, your exercise and your mind vary a great deal from week to week, even from day to day.

Make a simple graph to show you your pattern for the month. Plot the graph every day when you've completed your body diary by summing up how you felt on that day, taking everything you've written into account. It should range from 'terrible' to 'excellent'. For instance, on page 26 our example's Day 5 would rate as a 'good'. Her Day 26 would rate as a 'poor'.

For many women, a pattern will emerge that coincides with the stages of their monthly menstrual cycle. The cycle can, broadly, be divided up into three 'phases' as follows:

PHASE ONE: Beginning on day two or three of the menstrual period for most women, this is likely to be the **high-key phase**. At this phase, your body's levels of the hormone oestrogen gradually increase as you head towards ovulation when an egg is released from your ovaries. Most women find this is the phase at which they find it easiest to control their eating patterns and can use this as their best time to shed body fat as they are likely to feel happier on a reduced-calorie diet.

Mood is likely to be positive and temperament cool. The body should be 'running smoothly' and strength and stamina gradually build up in this phase, culminating in ovulation, which will be approximately 14 days from the start of your next period. For the two days around ovulation, for most women, their **high-key phase** will be at its peak. Research shows that this is when you are likely to feel least hungry, and your body to be at its strength peak coinciding with the highest levels of oestrogen in your body. Around ovulation you are also likely to feel creative, and your sex drive may increase.

PHASE TWO: Begins straight after ovulation, on or around Day 15 (assuming Day 1 to be the third day of your period). Once the egg is released into the fallopian tubes in its way towards the uterus (womb) and your body's oestrogen levels begin to decrease rapidly, your levels of another female hormone, progesterone, begin to increase and the uterus lining thickens in preparation for pregnancy. Appetite gradually increases throughout this phase. And body temperature and metabolic rate may rise.

Mood is often neutral or variable but energy and motivational levels should be high. Sex drive may continue to increase and strength and stamina potential is still good. Phase Two could be called the **neutral phase**.

PHASE THREE: Begins up to one week before your next period starts – for women on a regular 28-day cycle this would be around Day 20 or later. When your body realises that your egg hasn't been fertilised, progesterone production slows down dramatically and the womb lining is shed as your menstrual period. The first few days of Phase Three, before your period begins, are likely to be the days when you feel at your hungriest and appetite may be hard to control. You may feel hotter than usual; breast size may increase and you may gain weight temporarily, particularly around the stomach, due mainly to fluid retention.

At the end of this phase, when the period is beginning, the premenstrual symptoms reduce rapidly and, on or around Day 2 of your period, Phase One begins again.

The good news is that for most women, Phase Three can be 'managed' with the self-help methods that you will learn in

Bodysense. Appetite can be controlled, fluid retention and weight gain minimised, mood enhanced . . . with proper management, Phase Three – the **low-key phase** – can be as positive as any other time of the cycle in its own way.

Bodysense is largely about using these phases to help you slim, get fit and stay that way naturally.

Now here are the answers to the questions you will be asking:

'I have irregular periods – sometimes one every three weeks, other times I can go six weeks. Can I still use the three-phase system?'

Yes. Using your body diary to help you to spot changes, simply tune in to your body signals and choose the appropriate diet phase and exercise that most closely matches the way you feel on any particular day. Even if you have irregular periods, you will still experience different phases. I provide, in the chapters ahead, an eating plan for each phase – it is up to you to decide which phase you are on at any given time and how long to stay on it. For instance, with a longer-than-normal cycle, you may find you can stay on Phase One eating plan for three weeks or more; with a shorter cycle you may be on it for only a week or 10 days.

'I am on the Pill. Do the three phases apply to me?'

The Pill tends to 'flatten out' the effect of the three phases. Many women find Pre-menstrual syndrome (PMS) symptoms are less, that periods are lighter and that therefore the difference between the phases is not so noticeable. However, for most women on the Pill, there will still be a difference. Keep your month-long diary and see for yourself. If you are someone who doesn't notice much of a difference between the three phases because of the Pill, I suggest that you choose Phase Two eating plan for most of the time and on days when you feel strong and positive, change to Phase One.

'I don't have periods because I had a full hysterectomy. Can I still follow the *Bodysense* plan?'

The *Bodysense* plan – both eating and exercise – is extremely healthy and appropriate for you to follow. I suggest you choose Phase Two eating for most of the time and, on days when you feel strong and positive, change to Phase One. Keep Phase Three eating in reserve for things such as holidays, eating out, entertaining, and so on, as it allows you more to eat.

'I am pregnant. Should I still follow *Bodysense*?'

Specific advice for *Bodysense* during pregnancy appears in Chapter Eight. Please read that before beginning either the *Bodysense* eating or exercise plan.

'I am in the middle of my menopause. Can I still follow *Bodysense*?'

Yes you can. Keep your body diary, learn to read your body signals and choose the appropriate eating plan and exercise for whichever phase you appear to be on (using the guideline descriptions on pages 27–28). More advice for you during the menopause appears in Chapter Eight.

'I am 60 and my periods ceased several years ago. Is there any point in my following the *Bodysense* plan?'

The diet – in all its phases – is a very healthy one and you can follow it to lose weight. I suggest you use Phase Two eating for most of the time and Phase One on days when you feel like eating a little less. If, like many women, you have put yourself and your body last for many years, keeping the body diary will be very useful for you to get back in tune with its needs and 'ups and downs'. Even if we don't have periods, our bodies still do fluctuate and it is important, especially if you want to lose weight, to get in touch with these changes.

Every woman – whether she has periods or not – will find 'up' phases like Phase One, 'low-key' phases like Phase Three and 'just coasting along' phases like Phase Two in their lives. Learn to distinguish them for lifelong weight and fitness control.

· *Body Kindness* ·

So now you can see that it makes little sense to do what millions of women have done for many decades – tried to force their bodies to follow a day-in, day-out, week-in, week-out, diet régime that takes no account of the body's changing patterns.

And remember it is not just the menstrual cycle that affects your body.

Everything in your life interacts to produce the end effect – how you feel on any particular day. The dominant factor may well be the menstrual cycle, but you also need to consider what else is happening in your life – which is why your body diary is so useful.

For example, you may land a fabulous new job. On the day you learn about this, you are in Phase One of your cycle. That, coupled with your good news, conspires to give you, and your body, a *huge* high – you feel marvellous. However, suppose you learn the same news on a Phrase Three day when you got up feeling very low key? The new will probably turn your low-key phase into a Phase Two, or even a Phase One, feeling. Because it isn't just our hormones that govern how we feel – it is our emotions and life events, too.

That is why when you look at your body diary you may find 'mini-fluctuations' during a particular phase.

Here's another example. You meet someone and fall in love. In the first few weeks or months you may be on a near-permanent Phase One – your normal hormone patterns completely over-ridden by the adrenalin, endorphins and extra hormones that being in love can produce! Again, be kind to your body and use *this* prolonged 'Phase One' for weight control and a fitness régime.

Of course, life rarely consists of constant job promotions, falling in love, or, at the other end of the scale, tragedies and major setbacks. For most of us, these things happen from time to time, but for the greater part of our lives, things are more mundane; life is on more or less an even keel. Then your natural body phases will be the ones to which you pay most attention. So:

- Learn to read your body's signals. (The major signals will be linked to your menstrual periods.)
- Take into account what is happening in your life as this has a bearing on how you feel.

With a little practice, you can learn to spot your phases and use them to advantage in many areas of your life, not just for slimming, weight control and fitness. For example, knowing that the time around ovulation is one of great energy and creativity, you might organise a special meeting with a new client to discuss your ideas – or you might write that short story for a competition you want to enter! If you know that, for you, Phase Three brings an urge to tidy the house and get up to date with chores, leave them until then and get on with more important things for the rest of the month.

Bodysense will show you in the chapters ahead how to harmonise with yourself; how to tap into your own resources so that you enhance and use your 'highs' and minimise and manage your 'lows'. In this way you harness your body's natural energy and use it to the maximum.

You are going to tune into your body and stop asking it to behave in the same way all the time without complaining. You will lose weight the only sensible way – by making use of the days when you are capable of losing weight well, and by marking time during those days when you are not.

You are going to forget all about hopping on the bathroom scales every day. Indeed, one of the few rules of *Bodysense* is that you *don't* weigh yourself more than once a month so that you get a true picture of what weight you have really lost.

Remember – you don't want to fight; you want to be in tune with your body. That is when you will really be winning.

In the rest of the chapter we will look at body kindness in more detail.

· *Give Your Body Good Food* ·

Remember the saying, 'You are what you eat'? Whether you are slimming or weight maintaining, your body will work better for you – and, indeed, slim better for you – if you give it the nutrients it needs, when it needs them. Here are some of the ways that you can be kind to your body naturally, through food.

The first rule of good slimming is: give yourself enough food! The first thing most women do when they decide to lose weight is to cut themselves down to starvation rations – giving themselves tiny portions, often cutting out meals or replacing real food with things like shakes, energy bars or diet soups.

Or they will try one sort of crazy fad diet or another – like Melanie's citrus diet at the beginning of this chapter. None of these diets offers enough nutrition.

The only guaranteed way to *fail* on your diet is to eat too little. Women, even more than men, were not meant to go hungry. You may manage it for a few days, or even a couple of weeks, but no longer. Then you hit a Phase Three type of time – and you binge! So the rule of *Bodysense* eating is – when your body wants food, feed it! This is crucial to your success, and particularly in managing Phase Three when it is natural for you to want to eat more.

Yes, you *do* need to reduce your overall calorie intake over the months ahead in order to lose weight. The only alternative to that is to 'up' your calorie expenditure – i.e., the amount of calories you burn off in activity to create a deficit that way – but that, on its own, is a very slow way to slim indeed.

Research proves that it is the women who reduce their calorie intake by a small amount – and who choose good, wholesome food – who have the most success with long-term weight loss.

So, by refusing to keep your body hungry you are not only being kind to it, you are also making life easier for yourself and your diet too.

You will not lose masses of weight in a short space of time, but it doesn't matter because doing that has been proved to be unkind to your body.

What you will do is lose weight over the course of each month in a way that is right for you. You will use Phase One times to get into top gear with your slimming campaign since these are the times when you feel least hungry and can cope with slightly fewer calories than at other phases. You will also be burning up some extra calories with increased activity at all times of the month.

Combine the small reduction in calories with the increase in burning them off through exercise – and most women will see a monthly reduction in weight of around 2.3kg (4–6lbs) – quite naturally and without pain!

Is your body signalling hunger?

To keep your body satisfied with calories – and with nutrients – you need to learn to satisfy hunger with just enough – but no more. For most of us this is one of the hardest lessons to learn, as we are used to eating for all manner of reasons apart from natural hunger. Through habit we put too much food on our plates, we eat just because food is there; because advertisers have persuaded us to, and so on.

One key to succeeding this time is to get back in touch with your body's real hunger signals so that you eat when you are hungry and stop eating – or don't eat – when you are not.

Hunger pangs: a slight lightness in the lower abdomen; a rumbly tummy; increased sensitivity to food aromas and sights; thinking about food even when not reminded of it by seeing it.

You can also gauge hunger by how long it is since you last ate – if it is several hours *and* you have one or more of the above symptoms, then your hunger is probably justified, so eat.

Feelings that you may confuse with hunger: **boredom** – wanting something to do, so food comes to mind. **Habit** – you always sit down in front of the TV with some nuts and a drink; you don't think about whether you are hungry, you just do it. **Comfort** – you don't like whatever situation you are in, and food seems like a comforter. You could be in the middle of writing a difficult letter, so food seems like a good distraction – or you could have left your partner and are wondering whether you did the right thing. **Cravings** – feeling very strongly that you need a particular food, often chocolate or bread or any sweet food.

Go over your body diary and see if you can spot the things you ate not through hunger but for other reasons. Try to become aware every day of why you eat what you eat. This is the way to get back in tune with your real appetite.

The question of cravings will be dealt with in more detail in Chapter Three – but for now let me just say that if you eat correctly, the *Bodysense* way, cravings like these should disappear, especially if they are cravings that mostly appear in Phase Three.

Apart from simply being aware of eating for reasons other than real hunger, there are various things you can do to help to control your appetite so that you create a calorie deficit without eating too little. Here are some of my favourite ways:

- Put on your plate *more* of the high-bulk, lower-calorie items than usual and slightly less of the others. For instance, increase your portions of fresh vegetables, rice, pasta or potatoes, and decrease the amount of any fatty foods.
- If you end the meal still feeling genuinely hungry then you can always serve yourself a little more.
- When you have finished what is on your plate, stop for a couple of minutes. Take a drink of water, or similar. Do you still feel hungry? Probably not.
- Eat slowly. People who eat slowly have been shown to feel full on less than people who eat quickly.
- Don't let yourself get so hungry that you overeat when you *do* sit down for a meal. Which brings me on to the next point . . .

Give your body food at the right times

Most women have hungry times of day. A lot of women override their natural hungry times because they feel they will achieve quicker slimming success by doing so; or because they think their hungry times of day aren't convenient.

Then they wonder why they have problems with their weight and their appetite! To be kind to your body, you need to give it food when it wants it.

Many women quite naturally feel hungry soon after they get up in the morning – hardly surprising as the body has been on a 'fast' for 12 hours or more. Many of us are too rushed in the mornings to satisfy that hunger, so then we end up feeling ravenous by mid-morning – and eat totally unsuitable, unhealthy foods like biscuits and cakes.

Other people who have to get up early in the morning and have their breakfast early, will then have lunch early, and a meal early in the evening – only to find themselves ravenous just before bedtime, and pigging out in the kitchen on anything they can lay their hands on.

And then there are the people who have lunch at the regular time – 1pm – and their evening meal at the regular time – between 7pm and 8pm, and wonder why they get starving around 4 or 5 in the afternoon, and will end up snacking on biscuits or crisps or nuts while they are getting the children's tea, or preparing their own evening meal.

All situations such as these can ruin a slimming effort. And no wonder.

The fact is that for most of us, three meals a day are not enough. And if you are slimming, they are definitely not enough. The next fact is that all of the above situations can be controlled and rectified using the *Bodysense* plan, which allows your body a kind three meals a day plus two snacks *and* provides you with the types of foods that will help to keep hunger pangs at bay for longer. In the next chapter I will be showing you how this all works so that, even in the latter stages of Phase Two and all through Phase Three, you can control your appetite.

You will eat *more* than on conventional slimming diets, but in the end, you will achieve *more* success – and lose weight just as quickly – because overeating the wrong foods will become just a memory.

Give your body good exercise

Do you feel sluggish? Do you feel tired? Do you feel all tensed up – especially around the neck and shoulders? Listen to your breathing – are you, at this moment, virtually holding your breath, rather than breathing naturally? Are you finding it hard, really hard, to keep your weight under control although you don't really eat any more than you used to? Do you suffer from pre-menstrual cramps, constipation, fluid retention or sleeplessness?

If you can answer 'yes' to even one of those questions – and most of us will answer yes to many of them – then your body is crying out for some good exercise. Yes, now, as you are reading this.

Again, your body is giving you signals that you are choosing to ignore.

Your body is an exercise machine; it is there to move and lift and bend, stretch and walk and run, climb and burn energy. Exercise is one of the best natural tonics you can give your body and without it your body behaves just like an old rusty car in dire need of servicing and oiling. Without it, we get out of sorts and run sluggishly instead of efficiently – and we get overweight.

When we exercise, our bodies and minds work better. Exercise really is a near-miracle worker, especially for women.

We'll be working on your own exercise programme – which will take you as little as two hours a week, in Chapters Six and Seven. Don't skip them – if you want to be kind to your body, you can't afford to miss them out.

Respond to your body's needs

Eat for your body, exercise for your body – and give it consideration in every way that you can.

Use your body diary to consider, every day, how it feels and what you can do to put right anything that needs putting right. Consider how to de-stress yourself, how to cut down your workload; how to ease tiredness; how to get times of peace and quiet. Your body is a powerhouse if you let it be.

Food, sleep, activity, relaxation, leisure, stimulation – these are all sources of power that you can input. So *do* put them in – and just see what you get back in return.

3

FOOD AND BODYSENSE

In Chapter Two, you learnt that to lose weight naturally, you need to give your body good food, at the right times, and in the right quantities. This chapter provides you with all the information you need to do just that. You will learn:

- Which foods can make slimming harder and are best limited or avoided, especially at certain times.
- Which foods can make slimming easier by reducing hunger pangs and food cravings.
- How snacking is positively good for you.
- Why a very low-fat diet is unlikely to help you to achieve long-term slimming success.

And much more.

· *You Are What You Eat* ·

So that you can easily understand what I'm going to tell you about food and your slimming campaign, it's necessary for me to give you a two-minute rundown on the basics of 'good nutrition' – i.e., the basic eating recommendations from the Department of Health and the World Health Organisation (WHO) for a healthy diet, whether you are slimming or not.

The food that we eat is made up of a mixture of protein calories, carbohydrate calories, fat calories (and alcohol calories, if you drink), plus water, non-starch polysaccharides (fibre) and trace elements such as vitamins and minerals.

Good nutrition is about getting the right balance of all those things in our diets (except alcohol, which we don't actually need at all!). Very, very few foods contain just one of the above elements;

most contain a mixture. For instance, cheese is usually classed as a 'protein' food, but in fact, most cheeses contain much more fat than they do protein. Potatoes are thought of as a carbohydrate food, but also contain protein, and a tiny amount of fat. And so on.

Our diet today, in general, tends to contain *more* protein than we need; not *enough* carbohydrate of the right kind, and too *much* fat of the wrong kind; probably not enough *water*, too little *fibre* and some of us don't get enough of all the vitamins and minerals.

To alter the balance to a more suitable diet, what we need to do is this:

- Cut the fat in our diets by eating *fewer* high-fat protein foods such as Cheddar, Stilton, cream cheese, full fat milk and fatty cuts of meat, and replace most of them with low-fat protein foods such as pulses (dried beans, peas and lentils), fish, poultry and vegetable proteins like tofu.
- To make up the calorie deficit caused by eating less fat and a little less protein, we should eat *more* carbohydrate foods such as bread, potatoes, pasta, rice and other grains and pulses. (Pulses are the only foods to provide an almost perfect balance of protein, carbohydrate and fat in one package.)
- When cutting fat, we should try to cut down on *saturated* fat, found in largest quantities in high-fat dairy produce and meat.
- When eating carbohydrate, we should eat more *complex* carbohydrates, such as whole grains, pulses, fruits and vegetables, rather than *simple* carbohydrates such as sugar, sweets, confectionery and highly processed baked goods.
- We should eat plenty of fresh fruit and fresh vegetables.
- And to satisfy thirst, we should drink more water.

Following these guidelines, we would be eating the kind of diet deemed healthy by both the World Health Organisation and the Department of Health. And, indeed, the diet and menus in *Bodysense* do ensure that you eat in this way.

But for people wanting to watch their weight – or, indeed, lose weight – this 'healthy eating' pattern is not the end of the story. It is only the beginning.

For, within those guidelines, there is plenty we can do to make a slimmer's or weight-watcher's life a happier and an easier one.

And for women, this is particularly true.

What we will do is make minor refinements to a typical healthy diet.

Food, slimming and Bodysense

The fact is that some foods are more important in helping you to slim (or maintain a slim weight) than others. And, for women, certain types of food take on greater or lesser importance at certain phases.

First of all, let's look at the foods that keep hunger pangs at bay.

Nine women out of 10 who tell me that they have failed to lose weight and/or keep it off, say that they cannot control their hunger pangs.

'I can't stand that feeling of never quite having enough in my tummy to satisfy me.'

'When I am trying to slim, I suffer terrible hunger pains all evening.'

'It's all very well intending not to eat between meals, but when you are starving hungry, sooner or later, you're going to, aren't you?'

'I'm okay until I get anywhere near food, then I can't stop my hand going out and taking something and putting it in my mouth. Once I've done that – I can't stop.'

'The smell or the sight of the foods that I love – and which are banned – is just too much for me.'

Obviously, then, if you can discover a way of eating that dispenses with these hunger pangs and cravings, then you are going to be happy, and stick with the weight-loss plan for as long as it takes.

And this is what the *Bodysense* eating plan in Chapter Four provides: a way of eating that is not only beyond reproach health-wise, but that is also kind to your body. This is how it works.

● You will eat foods – and combinations of foods – that satisfy your appetite both in the short term and for longer . . . . particularly at the phases in your cycle when you need to do so most.

Appetite – and food cravings – are very strongly linked with your body's blood sugar levels. Usually the hungrier you feel, and/or the longer it is since you ate, the lower the levels of glucose (available energy) in your blood become. Low blood sugar levels can result in your feeling faint, dizzy, weak, sick and, usually, desperate for something to eat.

The 'something' that most people will eat will be something that is going to be quickly absorbed through the mouth and into the bloodstream – and that something is a 'simple carbohydrate', like sugar.

But this is just exactly the wrong thing to eat because it has the effect of stimulating the production of insulin in the body which can leave a residue, causing the blood sugar levels to plummet. . . . so, lo and behold, you crave *more* to eat and are likely to choose the wrong food again, and start the whole spiral off again.

What you need to do instead is keep that blood sugar level as constant as you can throughout the day, thus avoiding the hunger pangs and cravings that are so common in those on a diet.

'Ah, but!' I can hear lots of you saying now, 'I don't eat sugar; I know all about blood sugar levels and I make sure I eat a piece of bread instead, or some dried fruit.'

And this, you see, is where so many of us go wrong. Because bread and many types of dried fruit have just the same effect on your blood sugar levels as a spoonful of sugar!

Let me explain. Going back to that official healthy eating advice, to eat more 'complex' carbohydrates and less 'simple' carbohydrates. This sensible advice is based on the fact that 'complex' carbohydrates – the starchy foods like rice, pasta, potatoes, bread, grains and pulses – contain more fibre and more nutrients such as vitamins and minerals – than the 'simple' carbohydrates, particularly sugar-based products like sweets and biscuits.

Another distinction we should make between carbohydrates is how quickly they are absorbed into your bloodstream once you have eaten them, and how quickly they cause your blood sugar levels to rise.

Sugar, as we've already seen, causes a rapid rise in blood sugar levels, and therefore you can rightly assume that it is absorbed quickly into your bloodstream after being eaten.

But here is the amazing thing. Many of the 'complex' carbohydrate foods – and many fruits and vegetables – are also very quickly absorbed, causing a rapid blood sugar rise. Carrots, rice, most breads, including wholemeal, many breakfast cereals, including bran and muesli, baked potatoes, bananas – these are all carbohydrates that are absorbed quickly into your blood and have the same effect as sugar, causing a rapid return of hunger pangs!

The carbohydrates that are absorbed *slowly* into your bloodstream, keeping hunger pangs at bay for a long time, are again, not necessarily the ones you would expect and include apples, grapefruit, yogurt, and fructose (fruit sugar).

In between the two extremes are many foods that are absorbed neither rapidly nor slowly – the 'moderate' foods, such as pasta and oats.

So now you can begin to see how important it is – particularly at your 'hungry times' (such as before a period) to keep your blood sugar levels constant – and your appetite satisfied and hunger pangs at bay – with the right 'mix' of carbohydrates.

Other factors will also affect how quickly or slowly a carbohydrate is absorbed. Both fats and proteins release their energy slowly into your bloodstream, and so a 'quick release' carbohydrate food, eaten with a little fat or protein, will in effect become a slower-release food.

Because the rate at which food's energy is absorbed into the body is so important – not only in controlling blood sugar levels for slimmers, but also for sportspeople, for diabetics, and so on, scientists have devised an index, called the Glycaemic Index, rating each food with a Glycaemic Index number. Glucose (very rapidly absorbed) is given a GI of 100 and the nearer a food is to the 100 mark, the higher its GI is. For instance, white rice has a GI of 82 (high), oats have a GI of 49 (medium) and grapefruit has a GI of 26 (low).

That is not to say, though, that all foods with a high GI are bad and should be avoided. They provide instant energy, and that is something that can be a *good* thing (for instance for replenishing athletes' energy quickly during competition) but for slimmers, the secret is to balance your meals and snacks so that there is enough of the medium- and slow-release foods to offer both short-term satisfaction and long-term sustenance, and to compensate for the reduction in calories.

And this is the basis of the *Bodysense* diet. The eating plans in the next chapter have been worked out for you to provide that balance so that you needn't, in practice, worry too much about the GI of foods. But for your information a GI 'round up' of common foods is given below.

High Glycaemic Index foods (quick-release, instant energy)
Glucose, sugar, honey.
Baked potatoes, mashed potatoes, parsnips, cooked carrots, squash.
White rice, brown rice, wholemeal bread, white bread, rice cakes, bread sticks.
Cornflakes, branflakes, Weetabix, Shredded Wheat, muesli, instant oats, puffed cereal, popcorn, wheat crackers, muffins, crumpets.
Orange squash, watermelon, raisins, dried dates, Lucozade, sweetened yogurt, bananas.

Medium Glycaemic Index foods (moderate-release, mid-term energy)
Sweet potatoes, boiled potatoes, yam, raw carrot, sweetcorn.
White pasta, wholegrain pasta, oats, old-fashioned porridge, oatmeal biscuits, grapenuts, All-Bran, noodles.
Wholegrain rye bread, Ryvita, pitta bread, diabetic cookies.
Grapes, kiwifruit, mango, beetroot, fresh dates, figs, apple and date bars, rich tea biscuits.

Low Glycaemic Index foods (slow-release, long-term energy)
Baked beans, butter beans, chick peas, haricot beans, kidney beans, lentils, soya beans.
Barley, buckwheat, bulgar, couscous.
Apples, apricots, peaches, grapefruit, plums, oranges, cherries, orange juice.
Avocado, courgette, spinach, peppers, onions, mushrooms, spring greens, leeks, peas, green beans, sprouts, mangetout, broccoli, cauliflower.
Ice-cream, plain yogurt, milk.

Another look at protein and fat

Although, as we've seen, foods that contain no carbohydrate are not included on the Glycaemic Index, both fat and protein act like 'slow-release' carbohydrate foods in that they are slowly absorbed into the bloodstream and also have the effect of slowing down the absorption of the high GI foods. Thus, if you eat, say, a slice of white bread with a little sunflower margarine on it, it will turn into a medium-release snack.

So fat is very useful in the *Bodysense* diet. Used in small quantities, the right types of fat will help to keep you feeling satiated for longer. I say 'the right types of fat' because, although *all* fat has this slowing-down effect, for your health you should severely limit your intake of saturated fats, and whenever possible use monounsaturated fats, such as olive oil and groundnut oil, and high polyunsaturated fats such as corn oil.

Of course, fat is not just found in oil and butter. Nuts and seeds are useful sources of mono- and polyunsaturated fats. Oily fish such as salmon and mackerel are the main source of 'omega 3' type polyunsaturated fats which offer important protection against heart disease and strokes.

So *Bodysense* makes full use of these 'healthy fats', not only to help you to stick to your diet and make it more pleasant, but to help you to stay healthy, too.

All fats and oils, whether saturated or unsaturated, are high in calories though, so the art of using fat in your diet is to use just enough to reap benefit but not so much that you can't lose (or maintain) your weight.

· *Good Habits That Will Help to* · *Control Appetite*

Snacking

How many times do you hear people who are trying to lose weight say, 'I'm being very good; I'm sticking to mealtimes and not snacking. . .'

Fair enough, if your idea of snacking between meals is to eat a couple of chocolate bars and a packet of crisps then, yes, surely cutting those out will help you to lose weight.

But giving up snacking altogether is one of the worst things you can do.

For example, if you eat lunch at, say 1pm and then go until 7.30 or 8pm until your evening meal (which many busy women do) your stomach is going to be requesting food long before you get anywhere near that time of evening. Even after a slow-release lunch of, say, hummus and pitta bread with side salad, followed by a yogurt and an apple, there are only so many hours that that food will manage to keep your blood sugar constant. Eventually it will begin to dip, and at first you will exercise willpower and stop yourself grabbing at the biscuit tin – but by 6pm or so you'll give in.

Remember what I told you in Chapter Two? Be kind to your body. Give it something to eat before it gets to that stage.

And what you will give it is a 'best-mix' snack, again containing an optimum mix of quick- and slow-release carbo-hydrates with a tiny amount of fat and some protein.

In the next chapter you will learn all about best-mix snacks, and on the *Bodysense* eating plan you will be snacking, happily, on at least two of these satisfying snacks a day.

At no time do you have to go more than a couple of hours without something to eat. It's crucial!

Another poor time of day for many women is around 11.30am to 12 noon. We get up, rush around organising home and maybe family, catching up on chores, and grab a bowl of cereal if we're lucky, or a couple of slices of toast and marmalade before rushing off to work. After what, for most people, is a high GI breakfast (look back at that list and see just how many of your breakfast regulars *are* high GI), maybe we leave home at 8.30 or so. Lunch may not be until 1pm. But the after-effects of that toast are telling by 11; the blood sugar, having risen rapidly, is dipping rapidly and making you feel you could kill for a doughnut.

Here again, your best-mix snack comes to the rescue. (But of course, on *Bodysense,* your breakfast will have been a sensible mix of high and low GI foods so that, in any case, you're nowhere near as ravenous at 11am as you used to be.)

You begin to see?! *Bodysense* eating really does work.

Breakfast

We've mentioned breakfast but let's discuss here just how important breakfast is.

And for the slimmer, it *is* important. Let's say your evening meal is finished by around 8pm or a little later. You're cutting calories a little as you want to lose some body fat, so your evening meal is satisfying but in no way gargantuan. You go to bed, get up next morning and if you skip breakfast, is it any wonder you crave something sweet around 11am or even earlier? Your body cannot go 12 hours without food, and not complain about it.

Your body needs feeding soon after you get up in the morning to restore its blood sugar levels and help you to face the day.

If you can't face a large breakfast it doesn't matter all that much. You have to be kind to your body and give it what it wants. If it wants nothing more than cereal and fruit, then that is all right, as long as the cereal you choose is not one of the very high GI ones, and on the *Bodysense* eating plans all breakfasts listed are ones that provide plenty of 'slow release' and will sustain you until your next meal or snack.

Regular meals

Eating *regularly* is extremely important. Meals or snacks spaced out fairly evenly throughout the day are crucial to the success of your plan.

Again, along with the meals that are balanced to give you plenty of slow-release energy, regularly spaced meals are a safeguard against low blood sugar and hunger. And you will not suffer from food cravings for a chocolate bar or a piece of bread and honey.

The *Bodysense* eating plan should eliminate *all* uncontrollable food cravings and that includes pre-menstrual cravings, the Phase Three kind that are hardest to resist. Here's how.

· *The Three Stages of the Bodysense* · *Eating Plan*

As we saw in Chapter Two, most women's bodies and emotions are not constant. We change, from day to day, week to week, and the most common reason for this is the hormones that control our monthly cycle.

Because most diet plans ignore these fluctuations they are almost doomed to failure, because if you don't take account of these changes, problems such as bingeing, cravings and hunger will make you give up on the diet. So, the *Bodysense* plan is divided into three sections. Each section is based on mainstream, healthy eating (nothing faddy or cranky) but each phase matches your physical and emotional needs. The three plans go along with your body; they don't fight it. This is merely common sense.

Phase One

This is from around day 2 of your period until the end of ovulation in mid-cycle. This period of approximately two weeks for most women is when you are in 'top gear' and can make full use of your positivity, energy levels and reduced interest in food to do some serious slimming.

Because this is the time when appetite is most easily controlled, the Phase One eating plan supplies you with around 1,250 calories a day consisting of three meals and two small snacks. This is the lowest level of calories I would recommend any woman to eat on any long-term diet. Because the Phase One plan is very high in fruit and vegetables with the accent on fresh tastes and delicious meals, and because there are enough slow-release foods in the diet, you should find it easy to stick to this calorie level.

Phase Two

This is the 'neutral' time, lasting for around a week after the end of Phase One, when you may begin to notice, especially towards the end of the phase, that you are beginning to feel more hungry.

The Phase Two eating plan is geared to helping you to lose weight slightly less quickly than on Phase One, at around 1,400 calories a day, consisting of three meals and two best-mix snacks. The amount of moderate to low GI foods is gradually increasing so that we can still create a calorie deficit for you without your feeling hungry. The fat and protein content of your meals increases slightly, too.

Protein, latest research shows, is better than carbohydrate and even better than fat at helping to control your appetite. So, although protein only makes up around 15 per cent of your total calorie intake, it *is* important to ensure that you get regular supplies of protein in your *Bodysense* diet.

The main problem with much of the protein foods (meats and dairy produce) that we eat is that it is, typically, high in fat and particularly saturated fat, unless we deliberately choose the low-fat versions.

But other sources of protein contain either very little fat, or else the fat they do contain is not saturated.

Very low fat protein sources: Quorn, tofu, pulses, white fish, shellfish, game, TVP mince, low-fat yogurt, milk and fromage frais.

Unsaturated fat protein sources: Oily fish, nuts and seeds.

These are the proteins we should choose.

So, to sum up, the meals and snacks you eat on the *Bodysense* diet help you to feel satisfied and keep hunger pangs at bay for longer – because they contain an optimum mix of protein, fats and carbohydrates, and the carbohydrates will be the optimum mix and quantity of fast- medium- and slow-release carbohydrates according to the phase and other factors.

Phase Three

This is the pre-menstrual phase, lasting up to a week and until you are into day 2 or 3 of your period, when being kind to yourself really comes into its own. By eating the right types of food at the right time, and by doing the right exercise as detailed in Chapters Six and Seven, you can enjoy Phase Three very much.

It is the time at which your appetite is naturally greater than during the rest of the month and it is essential that you eat more food at this time to avoid cravings, binges or hunger.

To achieve this, the Phase Three eating plan provides a minimum of 1,600 calories a day, consisting of three meals and two satisfying best-mix snacks which keep your blood sugar levels constant throughout the day. On this calorie level, most women will, in theory, achieve a small fat loss of up to 225g (1/2 lb) in a week but, because of the natural tendency to put on weight at this time, this fat loss won't be apparent until Phase One begins again. (For more information on the pre-menstrual weight gain, see the following Q and A section.)

During Phase Three you should avoid alcohol and cut right back on simple carbohydrates such as sugary foods and drinks. And resist the temptation to hop on the scales.

The Phase Three plan is very high in the low GI foods, and fat and protein content increases a little.

· *Your Questions Answered* ·

I have very irregular periods, can I still use the *Bodysense* eating plans?

Yes, you can. The plans are suitable for all women, even if you don't have a regular cycle or, indeed, even if you don't have periods at all. All you do is follow these guidelines:

USE PHASE ONE eating plan on days when you feel strong, relaxed, upbeat, physically good and you aren't feeling particularly hungry.

If you do have periods, even if irregular, always begin the Phase One eating plan as soon as your period is well under way, usually on day 2 or 3, and keep on Phase One as long as you feel able to, then switch to Phase Two.

USE PHASE TWO eating plan on 'average' days, when things are ticking over and you feel in a neutral frame of mind. You can also use the Phase Two plan on days when you slot in more exercise than usual and you may need those extra calories.

USE PHASE THREE eating plan on days when you want to be extra kind to yourself. Everyone has days when they wake up and know they are going to have to work extra hard to get into gear. We also have days when we feel hungrier than other times. This is a Phase Three type of day, so follow the Phase Three eating plan.

I don't seem to have much variation in how I feel throughout my cycle. Is this unusual and can I still follow the *Bodysense* system?

Around 75 per cent of women confirm that they feel different at different times of the month and the *Bodysense* phases match their most common experiences and patterns.

But, of course, not everyone is typical and some women will feel much milder changes than others (particularly if you are on the pill).

If you are one of those women who feels little or no alteration in your needs, feelings, capabilities etc. throughout the month then I suggest, if you need to lose weight, that you start off on the Phase Two eating plan and see how you get on. This should result in steady weight loss. If then you find you're losing weight very slowly – say, less than 1–1.5kg (2–3lbs) a month, you could perhaps use Phase One eating plan to speed this up slightly, if you want to. Use Phase Three eating plan for days when you want extra food – e.g., if you are going out, entertaining, etc., or simply feel like a little extra.

I suffer badly from fluid retention before my period. Will the *Bodysense* eating plans help that at all?

A certain amount of fluid retention before a period is natural and normal and is the main cause of the weight gain so many women complain of at this time. It's unwise to try to eliminate this altogether and I wouldn't recommend diuretics, but you can help to keep it to a minimum with *Bodysense*.

Things that make fluid retention worse are a high salt diet, a high simple carbohydrate diet, and big meals. *Bodysense* avoids all those – and helps positively by encouraging you to eat the few foods that are naturally diuretic, such as fresh fruits and salad vegetables.

I suffer from constipation for a few days before every period. What can I do about this, as it makes me feel even fatter and more bloated, and does my morale no good at all.

You need to drink plenty of water (which, incidentally, *doesn't* cause extra fluid retention), eat lots of fresh fruit, especially citrus fruit, and lots of pulses and vegetables and certain dried fruits. The *Bodysense* Phase Three plan offers all this, already thought out for you.

It is also very important to take plenty of exercise – regular walking and swimming are both good at eliminating constipation.

Even if I follow a diet to the letter, I always put on 1.5–2kg (3–4lbs) before my period. It is very discouraging. Is there any way to stop this weight gain?

Happily this weight gain is not fat, but mostly fluid retention caused by hormones in your body and as soon as your period is well under way you will find yourself going to the loo more frequently and this extra fluid will be passed in your urine. Another cause for many women is constipation – if you suffer badly before a period you could put on 1–1.5kg (2–3lbs) through this alone. See the previous two answers for how to deal with these problems which, always remember, are temporary.

I sometimes get a bit depressed before my period and, even though I know what is causing these feelings, I feel the need to 'comfort' eat. So no matter how good I am at slimming for the rest of the month, I put back every pound that I've lost in those few days and after my period I have to start all over again. Have you any advice?

One of the main objectives of *Bodysense* is to help you to avoid bingeing in a Phase Three (pre-menstrual) phase, so I hope that when you try the *Bodysense* diet as described in this book, your urge to 'comfort' eat before your periods will disappear.

The even better news is that the *Bodysense* way of eating – a high starch diet, high in low Glycaemic Index foods – can actually relieve the symptoms of Pre-menstrual stress (PMS), including depression. So let's hope that not only your comfort eating, but your depression, too, may be cured!

I sleep very badly in the few days before my period and this makes me tired and irritable during the daytime and too weak-willed to stick to a diet. What can I do?

A drink of skimmed milk with a little low-fat malted drink in it should help you to sleep. Milk contains a substance which helps to calm you down. And/or you could try a herbal remedy – passionflower tablets work well for me (from health food shops and many chemists). Also remember the 'be kind to your body'

Bodysense philosophy at this time and make sure to follow the Phase Three eating plan, not One or Two. The extra calories and special menus during this phase will mean that you won't really *need* willpower anyway. Get back to serious slimming after day 2 or 3 of your period.

There are so many supplements advertised for women – for instance, calcium tablets, evening primrose oil, premenstrual combinations, and so on. Do I really need to take any of them?

The safest answer to that is that if you think you may need a supplement, talk through your worries with your doctor. If a supplement really is necessary – or worth trying – you can get it on prescription.

For example, evening primrose oil can be helpful in alleviating many PMS symptoms such as tender breasts. And calcium tablets are useful in supplementing the diets of women at risk of osteoporosis who aren't getting enough calcium in their normal diets.

But there is little point in 'treating' yourself with a supplement just on the off-chance it might do some good. If you are eating a healthy diet it is unlikely that you need vitamin supplements unless you are a 'special case' (a heavy smoker or drinker, pregnant, ill, suffering from stress. . .) and in all these cases you should see your doctor to discuss the right treatment for you.

Are there such things as 'superfoods' – foods that are almost perfect? And if so, what are they?

The main thing you need nutritionally is an overall varied diet, not a diet that relies too heavily on a few foods.

That said, there are some foods that do seem particularly beneficial such as broccoli (rich in fibre, vitamin C, iron, and the anti-oxidant beta-carotene and selenium *and* containing no fat or sugar with few calories per portion). Other well-blessed foods include lentils, soya beans, sweet potatoes, red peppers, to name a few.

But the main requirement of a 'superfood' is that it is enjoyable to eat. Remember that no 'superfood' is so brilliant that you can eat it as part of an unbalanced diet and stay healthy. The *Bodysense* eating plans make full use of the particularly beneficial foods but not to the exclusion of all else.

4

THE BODYSENSE DIET

Before you begin the plan in this chapter, make sure you've read Chapter Three thoroughly because it gives you all the background detail you need to know.

To sum up:

- The diet is in three phases. **Phase One** is your most active slimming phase suitable for days when you feel good and 'in control'. For most women this will relate to the two weeks directly after their period has begun. **Phase Two** is a moderate slimming phase, suitable for neutral days. For most women this will relate to the week following their ovulation in mid-cycle. **Phase Three** is the stage for being kind to yourself, when you aren't actively trying to lose weight but are giving your body the good, regular food that it needs in the right quantities and of the right types to help prevent PMS, hunger, bingeing and cravings. For most women, this will be the few days preceding their period and into the first day or two of their period, or at any time when under stress.

- The diet relies on:
  - Regular eating throughout the day, with a maximum of three hours between meals or snacks.
  - Plenty of moderate and low Glycaemic Index (GI) foods to keep blood sugar levels steady.
  - High intake of complex carbohydrates and low intake of simple carbohydrates.
  - High intake of fresh fruits and vegetables.
  - Low intake of saturated fats but overall fat content kept moderate rather than extremely low.

· *How and When to Begin the Diet* ·

If you are having periods, I suggest that you begin the plan on Day 3 of your period, using Phase One. Continue with this phase until immediately after ovulation (usually at mid-cycle), which . means you will be on Phase One for about two weeks.

How do you tell when you are ovulating? For most women, there is a sudden rise in body temperature at or just after ovulation. Many women experience a little mid-cycle pain in the lower abdomen on the ovulating side, lasting for a few minutes or intermittently over a few hours. And, research shows, women are at their strongest physically and at their peak of creative powers during the day or two around ovulation – so look out for these signs.

Straight after ovulation, move to Phase Two and stay on this until five to seven days before your period begins. Learn to listen to your body signals as we discussed in Chapter Two so that you can hear it telling you when you need to begin eating more – for instance, if you begin to feel hungry on Phase Two, or have any PMS symptoms, then you know it is time to move on to Phase Three. Once on Phase Three, stay on it until you are well into your period – about day 3. Then begin Phase One again.

If you don't have periods, follow the guidelines in Chapter Two for how best to use the phases. If you are pregnant, read the pregnancy section in Chapter Eight.

Each phase has a set, seven-day diet (which can be repeated to cover the number of days you want to stay on that phase). I suggest that everyone follows the set diets to begin with until you are well used to eating the *Bodysense* way. Under each phase are several pages of lunch and main meal suggestions so that you can expand your menu over the months ahead – choosing a lunch and an evening meal to suit yourself. Finally, for even more choice, you can use the food charts at the end of the book to devise your own diet, but it is best not to attempt this until you have followed the menus in this chapter for at least two months.

· *Weight Loss* ·

You should not think in terms of weekly weight loss but in terms of monthly weight loss. This is because your body naturally loses most weight in the two weeks after a period, and then, naturally, this slows down. I suggest that you weigh yourself at the end of Phase One every month – i.e., around ovulation time. I don't want to predict how much weight you will lose as, to be honest, I can't. This will be governed by several factors. For instance, the more overweight you are, the more weight you are likely to lose in a month. The more time you spend on Phase One and the less on Phase Three, the more you will lose in a month.

The one thing I can tell you is that the diet isn't geared to rapid weight loss. The most you should lose is around 4.5kg (9lb) a month. Most women – especially if you are over 40 – should be happy with a loss of around 2.5kg (5lbs) a month, a figure that should keep your body happy and keep you motivated. You will, of course, be doing some exercise (see Chapters Six and Seven) which will help, too.

· *Scales* ·

Don't weigh yourself every week. Weigh yourself once a month only. Our weight varies naturally at different times of the month (we usually weigh more before a period), so it makes no sense at all to jump on the scales and expect a weight loss at that time.

You will only be disappointed, perhaps feel a failure, and be more likely to overeat. Weigh yourself around mid-cycle, or at the end of a Phase One slimming plan.

· *Diet Instructions and Tips* ·

Every day throughout the *Bodysense* diet, in all phases, you have a **daily milk allowance** of 140ml (1/4 pint) skimmed milk, for use in tea and coffee or as a drink on its own. If you don't want this milk allowance, you should have a Shape yogurt or a few spoonfuls of low-fat natural yogurt instead, as you need the calcium, protein and nutrients.

Unlimited throughout all phases of the diet are: all salad greens and leafy green vegetables (raw or plainly cooked, as lightly as possible), water, mineral water, fresh herbs and spices; lemon juice.

Portion sizes are not given for most **vegetables** in the diet – you should eat large portions whenever you can. Sometimes I simply suggest which vegetables you should choose, but the final choice is up to you, and what is available. When choosing your own vegetables, make sure to get plenty of dark green, and orange- and red-fleshed ones for the vitamin C, beta-carotene and minerals they contain.

Most vegetables are low in calories but some are a little higher. Serve yourself medium portions of these higher calorie vegetables: sweetcorn, parsnips, peas, broad beans, beetroot.

Unless otherwise stated, all vegetables should be cooked plain, without added fat, and should never be overcooked.

· *Vegetarians* ·

Vegetarians can follow the diet – a veggie choice is given for every day on the set menu and the free choice meals contain a vegetarian selection too. I have also, whenever possible, given a vegetarian version of the recipe dishes in Chapter Five (see the 'tips' section under individual recipes).

As we discussed in the previous chapter, some carbohydrate foods, while being nutritionally good for you, have a high Glycaemic Index and thus don't satisfy your hunger or keep your blood sugar levels as constant as do the carbohydrates with a lower GI.

Both standard wholemeal and white **breads** have a fairly high GI. This is probably because the flour is ground so fine, even in wholemeal bread, that it passes quickly through your system. The breads that have a lower GI and are, therefore, better for the purposes of the *Bodysense* diet, are black rye bread, traditional stoneground wholemeal bread and wholegrain bread.

Choose these latter breads as often as you can in preference to white or mass-produced wholemeal. You can often buy black rye bread in delicatessens, health food shops and supermarkets.

If black rye bread is mentioned in the diet and you can't get it, substitute pitta or wholegrain.

Many breakfast **cereals** have a high GI and won't sustain you through a hard morning's work. The high GI cereals, which you should try to avoid, are: Cornflakes, Branflakes, Ready Brek, Puffed Wheat, Shredded Wheat and Rice Crispies.

There are plenty of alternatives, as you will see in the Breakfast section below.

All fresh **fruit** is good for you and you should eat plenty, but some fruits have a much higher GI than others. If eating fruit on its own as a snack, it is best to know which is which so that you can choose a lower GI fruit to help to stave off hunger pangs for longer. Sometimes within the diet I will state 'choose a low GI fruit' and then you can select from this list: apples, apricots, peaches, nectarines, grapefruit, plums, cherries, oranges.

Fruits with a very high GI are bananas and watermelon. Other fruits, such as grapes and fresh dates, are medium GI.

Some dried fruits also have a high GI so should be avoided as a hunger-staving snack on their own. These are raisins, sultanas and dried dates. All other dried fruits are medium GI.

· *Desserts* ·

It makes *Bodysense* to avoid desserts that are high in sugar, saturated fat and calories, and low in nutrients. Sweet toothers will almost certainly find their sweet tooth diminishing after a week or two of eating the *Bodysense* way, but remember that fruit is sweet and there will be plenty of sweet, satisfying snacks during the day.

The problem with traditional desserts, is that you eat them when you are not really hungry, and in *Bodysense*, as you've learnt, your food intake is spaced out evenly throughout the day. You eat when your body needs food, and you never eat more than you need. Think of your best-mix snacks as your alternative desserts – and if you're ever really longing for a sweet treat at the end of a meal, have some fruit.

· *Best Mixes* ·

In Phases Two and Three, mid-morning and mid-afternoon you will be asked to choose a best-mix snack. These are so called because they are an ideal mix of fast- and slow-release foods, including a little protein and very little fat. Choose from the following lists when you are asked to pick a best-mix.

Phase Two best mixes

- 50g (2 heaped tablespoons) 8% fat fromage frais (mixed with a little mustard or curry powder or tomato paste if you like) used as a dip with a selection of raw vegetables (e.g., peppers, spring onions, cauli florets) plus 1 dark rye Ryvita
- 1 no added sugar apple fruit bar; 1 plum
- 1 slice any melon except watermelon; 1 Shape diet yogurt; 1 Ryvita with a very little low-fat spread
- 15g (1/2 oz) reduced fat Edam cheese; 1 Ryvita; 1 kiwifruit
- 50g (2 heaped tablespoons) cottage cheese; 1 Ryvita; 1 apple
- 6 shelled almonds; 1 plum; 1 kiwifruit
- 1 savoury low salt oatcake; 1 small apple
- Fruit salad of 1 fresh or dried fig, 100g (3 1/2 oz) orange-fleshed melon, a 1/2 grapefruit with a little fructose and orange juice plus 1 dessertspoon 8% fat fromage frais
- Fruit salad of 1 apple, 50g (2oz) seedless grapes and 1 teaspoon sesame seeds in a little apple juice with 1 dessertspoon 8% fat fromage frais
- 2 dark rye Ryvitas, one with 1 teaspoon jam made with fructose (diabetic type), the other with 1 x 25g (1oz) slice extra lean ham.

Phase Three best mixes

- 50g (2 heaped tablespoons) low-fat cheese dip (see recipe on page 82) plus selection of raw vegetables plus 1 mini pitta
- 1 Breakfast Muffin (see recipe, page 83), 1 small apple; 75ml (3fl oz) skimmed milk
- 1/2 portion Pasta and Tuna salad (see page 104)
- 1/2 portion Cheese, Pineapple and Pasta salad (see recipe, page 106)

- ¹/₂ portion Mixed Bean Salad with Fruit (see recipe, page 106)
- 100g (3¹/₂ oz) reduced-salt, reduced-sugar baked beans on 1 medium slice dark rye toast; 1 plum or apricot
- 50g (2 tablespoons) hummus, 1 mini pitta; 1 orange
- 25g (1oz) All-Bran; 1 small banana, chopped, 75ml (3fl oz) skimmed milk, 1 teaspoon sesame seeds
- 50g (2oz) butter bean pâté (made by blending drained canned butterbeans with a little 8% fat fromage frais and seasoning) on 1 medium slice dark rye bread; 1 apple
- ¹/₂ portion Lentil Soup (see recipe page 80; 2 dark rye Ryvitas
- 2 savoury oat cakes; 1 small banana; 1 plum or 50g (2oz) cherries

· *Breakfasts* ·

Throughout all phases of the diet, choose *one* of the following breakfasts every morning. Try to vary your choices as much as possible.

Cereal breakfast

Choose one of the following:

- Medium bowl porridge (not the instant kind) made with water and 50ml (2fl oz) skimmed milk
- 40g (1¹/₂ oz) All-Bran
- 25g (1oz) grapenuts
- 25g (1oz) no added sugar luxury muesli

To your cereal, add 1 level tablespoon sunflower or sesame seeds.

Now add 1 portion of any fresh fruit you like *or* five ready-to-eat prunes or dried apricots and finally add 1 small tub natural low-fat Bio yogurt *or* 1 Shape diet yogurt *or* 140ml (¹/₄ pint) skimmed milk.

Baked bean breakfast

200g (7oz) low-sugar, low-salt baked beans in tomato sauce, heated, on 1 x 50g (2oz) slice dark rye bread, toasted, with a very little low-fat spread.

Follow with 1 portion of fresh fruit of your choice.

Fruit salad breakfast

- 1 portion Fruit and Nut Compote (see recipe, page 108) plus 125ml (4^1/$_2$ fl oz) skimmed milk *or* 2 tablespoons natural low-fat Bio yogurt
- 1 portion Cool Fruit Salad (see recipe, page 110) plus 100g (3^1/$_2$ oz) 8% fat fromage frais; 15g (^{1}/$_2$ oz) All-Bran; ^{1}/$_2$ slice dark rye bread with a very little low-fat spread.

Breakfast muffin

1 Breakfast Muffin (see recipe page 83) plus 1 chopped apple or 2 fresh apricots, chopped, in 2 tablespoons natural low-fat Bio yogurt. Follow with 1 small slice dark rye bread topped with 2 teaspoons pure fruit spread. You can use 125g (4^1/$_2$ oz) apple stewed with a little fructose instead if you like.

· PHASE ONE ·

The seven-day set diet

- The seven days can be repeated as necessary, as long as you are on Phase One. Once you are happy with following the programme, you can choose your lunches and evening meals from the free choices that follow on pages 65–67.

- Read all the instructions on pages 53–60 before beginning and don't forget your daily allowance of milk and your unlimited items, especially up to 8 glasses of water a day.

· Day One ·

Breakfast
Choose one from pages 59–60.

Mid-morning snack
Choose a low GI fruit from the list on page 57.

Lunch
Mushroom scramble: Spray a small saucepan with Fry Light. Add two eggs beaten with 2 tablespoons skimmed milk and seasoning, plus 50g (2oz) sliced mushrooms. Scramble over a medium heat and serve with a 40g (1¹/₂ oz) slice dark rye bread plus a large mixed salad with oil-free French dressing.

Follow with a diet fromage frais (e.g., Shape) and a small glass of orange juice.

Mid-afternoon snack
As mid-morning.

Evening meal
1 portion Chicken and Pasta Peperonata (see recipe, page 83)
or
100g (3¹/₂ oz) chicken breast fillet (no skin), baked in foil with seasoning, or microwaved, with one red pepper, sliced and stir-fried in 1 dessertspoon olive oil until the pepper is soft, plus 100g (3¹/₂ oz) new potatoes and broad beans or peas.

* *For vegetarians:* Serve the stir-fried pepper with 150g (5oz) cubed tofu stirred into it plus 1 dessertspoon light soya sauce, instead of the chicken.

· *Day Two* ·

Breakfast
Choose from pages 59–60.

Mid-morning snack
As Day One.

Lunch
50g (2oz) hummus with 1 wholemeal pitta (large), a large mixed salad with oil-free French dressing *or* 1 level tablespoon 70% fat-free mayonnaise, and 1 Shape diet yogurt.

Mid-afternoon snack
As Day One.

Evening Meal
One portion Baked Salmon and Rice with a Creamed Coulis (see recipe, page 89)
or
1 medium salmon fillet or steak, grilled, microwaved or poached (you can brush the salmon with a little French mustard if you like), plus 6 tablespoons cooked brown rice; mangetout or green beans and broccoli

**For vegetarians:* Make a 110g (4oz) burger out of cooked brown lentils bound with a little seasoned mashed potato and cook in a non-stick pan with Fry Light – or use a RealEat VegeBurger made from packet mix without the egg.

· *Day Three* ·

Breakfast
Choose from pages 59–60.

Mid-morning snack
As Day One.

Lunch
1 portion Baby Vegetable and Chicken Salad (see recipe, page 104
plus one medium banana.

(Vegetarians use 200g (7oz) mixed ready cooked beans in the
salad instead of the chicken.)

Mid-afternoon snack
As Day One.

Evening Meal
Couscous with a selection of roast vegetables: Soak 50g (2oz) dry-
weight couscous according to packet instructions, but using
vegetable stock instead of water. Keep warm. Chop a selection of
vegetables from this list: new potatoes, carrot, swede, squash,
parsnip, sweet potato, aubergine, courgettes, red pepper – into
medium chunks, brush with a little olive oil and roast for 45–50
minutes, turning once. Serve on the couscous and top with 2
tablespoons Parmesan cheese.

· *Day Four* ·

Breakfast
Choose from the list on pages 59–60.

Mid-morning snack
As Day One.

Lunch
Half a ripe avocado, sliced and mixed with 1 large sliced tomato, 2
chopped spring onions, mixed salad leaves, 25g (1oz) chopped
nuts, all tossed in oil-free French dressing and served with 2 dark
rye Ryvitas. 1 apple.

Mid-afternoon snack
As Day One.

Evening Meal
1 portion Lamb and Lentil Casserole (see recipe, page 97) served
with 2 tablespoons cooked brown rice or bulgar wheat.

*For vegetarians: follow the instructions for altering the recipe
on page 98.

· *Day Five* ·

Breakfast
Choose from the list on pages 59–60.

Mid-morning snack
As Day One.

Lunch
1 portion Pasta and Tuna Salad (see recipe, page 104. Vegetarians can omit the tuna and add 50g (2oz) extra beans and sweetcorn to the recipe.

Mid-afternoon snack
As Day One.

Evening Meal
Prawn omelette: Beat 2 size 3 eggs with a little seasoning and 1 tablespoon water; heat non-stick frying pan sprayed with Fry Light and when very hot add the eggs and make an omelette, adding 50g (2oz) prawns at the last minute. Fold and serve with 100g (3^1/$_2$ oz) new potatoes, a portion of peas and broccoli or a green vegetable of your choice.

For vegetarians: Use 1 tablespoon 8% fat fromage frais and 50g (2oz) chopped mushrooms blended into it, to fill your omelette.

· *Day Six* ·

Breakfast
Choose from the list on pages 59–60.

Mid-morning snack
As Day One.

Lunch
1 portion Lentil Soup (see recipe, page 80) with 1 medium slice dark rye bread

Mid-afternoon snack
As Day One.

Evening Meal
1 portion Tagliatelle with Mixed Vegetable Sauce (see recipe, page 84).

or

75g (3oz) dry weight tagliatelle, boiled and served topped with 5 tablespoons ready-made Italian tomato sauce plus 75g (3oz) sliced mushrooms and 1 extra tablespoon Parmesan cheese.

· *Day Seven* ·

Breakfast
Choose from the list on pages 59–60.

Mid-morning snack
As Day One.

Lunch
50g (2oz) half-fat hard cheese (e.g., Cheddar or Edam) with 1 medium banana, 1 apple, celery, 1 dessertspoon sweet pickle and 3 dark rye Ryvitas.

Mid-afternoon snack
As Day One.

Evening Meal
1 portion Turkey and Nut Stir Fry (see recipe, page 94).
  *For vegetarians: Use Quorn or tofu chunks instead of the turkey in the recipe.

Repeat the week to continue on Phase One or choose freechoice lunches and evening meals from the list below.

· *Phase One Freechoice Lunches* ·

Vary your choices as much as possible.

- Any lunch from the Phase One set diet.
- 1 portion Potato and Broccoli Soup (see recipe, page 82) with 1 x 50g (2oz) slice dark rye bread; 1 diet yogurt; 1 apple.
- 1 x 100g (3¹/₂ oz) pot cottage cheese; 3 dark rye Ryvitas with a little low-fat spread; 1 orange; 1 muffin (see recipe, page 83).
- 1 x 100g (3¹/₂ oz) slice vegetable terrine served with a large mixed salad and 1 x 50g (2oz) slice dark rye bread; 1 banana.

- 550ml (1 pint) fresh (from chilled counter) lentil and vegetable soup; 1 medium slice dark rye bread; 1 plum or fresh apricot.
- Half a medium avocado filled with oil-free French dressing, 3 dark rye Ryvitas; large mixed salad; 1 medium banana.
- Salad made from 6 tablespoons cooked leftover couscous mixed with 50g (2oz) cooked chick peas, a selection of chopped raw vegetables/salad items of choice (e.g., celery, tomato, peppers) and 25g (1oz) dried apricots, all tossed in oil-free French dressing; plus 1 x 50g (2oz) slice dark rye bread; 1 apple.
- 550ml (1 pint) fresh (from chilled counter) Tuscan Bean Soup with 1 medium slice dark rye bread; 1 medium banana.
- Open sandwich of 1 x 50g (2oz) slice dark rye bread topped with 50g (2oz) lean chicken meat and sliced tomato, onion and pepper plus half a small avocado, sliced. Drizzle oil-free French dressing over top *or* have 1 level dessertspoon 70% fat-free mayonnaise; 1 peach or nectarine or orange.
- 1 can Heinz Pea and Ham soup 300g (11oz) with 3 Ryvitas; 1 125ml (4¹/₂ fl oz) pot natural low-fat Bio yogurt with 1 large banana.
- 200g (7oz) can baked beans on 1 x 50g (2oz) slice dark rye bread; 1 orange.
- 200g (7oz) sliced mushrooms, stir-fried in 1 dessertspoon olive oil and served on 1 x 50g (2oz) slice dark rye bread with 2 tablespoons Parmesan cheese on top; 1 diet yogurt; 1 plum or kiwifruit.
- 3 dark rye Ryvitas each topped with 1 tablespoon low-fat cream cheese (e.g., Philadelphia Light) plus a selection of sliced salad vegetables; 1 apple and date bar; 1 orange.

· *Phase One Freechoice Evening Meals* ·

- Any Evening Meal from the Phase One Set Diet.
- Half pack mixed frozen seafood (usually prawns, mussels, squid) defrosted and simmered in 150ml (5¹/₂ fl oz) Italian tomato sauce and served with 75g (3oz) dry weight pasta of choice, boiled; large mixed salad.
- 1 portion Baked Salmon and Rice with a Creamed Coulis (see recipe, page 89); 1 portion mangetout or peas or green beans.

- 1 portion Salmon and Spinach Pie (see recipe, page 90); green salad.
- 1 portion Grilled Cod with a Tomato and Red Pepper Salsa (see recipe, page 90); 6 tablespoons cooked couscous *or* 200g (7oz) boiled potato; 1 portion baby sweetcorn or peas or broccoli.
- 1 portion Quick Sautéed Fish and Tomato Sauce (see recipe, page 91); 1 portion broccoli; 1 portion peas; 150g (5oz) boiled potato *or* 1 baked potato skin, quartered and baked until crispy.
- 1 portion Tuna Fish Cakes (see recipe, page 92); 1 portion spinach or other green vegetables; 1 portion peas and carrots; 1 apple.
- 1 portion Chilli Chicken (see recipe, page 96) served with 40g (1¹/₂ oz) dry weight egg thread noodles, cooked according to packet instructions; green side salad.
- 1 portion Chicken Tuscany (see recipe, page 97) served with 40g (1¹/₂ oz) dry weight pasta of choice, boiled, and 1 portion mangetout or broccoli.
- 1 large sweet potato, pricked and baked until tender, halved and served topped with 2 tablespoons grated Parmesan mixed with 2 tablespoons 8% fat fromage frais and seasoning; large mixed salad with 1 tablespoon of oil-free French dressing.
- 1 portion Pork and Pepper Stir Fry (see recipe, page 99) served with 50g (2oz) dry weight egg thread noodles, cooked according to packet instructions.
- 1 portion Mushroom Risotto (see recipe, page 99); green side salad.
- 1 portion Ratatouille and Eggs in a Baked Herb Crust (see recipe, page 100); plus 50g (2oz) dark rye bread.
- 1 portion Gratin of Pulses and Vegetables (see recipe, page 101); 5 tablespoons cooked brown rice or couscous.
- 1 large red pepper, topped and de-seeded and filled with 1 portion Spicy Rice Stuffing (see recipe, page 109); 1 diet fromage frais or yogurt.
- 1 small breast of chicken portion, grilled and skin removed; 1 medium sweet potato, baked; 2 portions green vegetables of choice.
- 1 lean pork stead, brushed with a little honey and soya sauce and grilled; 1 medium sweet potato, baked, two portions green vegetables of choice.

· *PHASE TWO* ·

The seven-day set diet

● The seven days can be repeated as necessary for as long as you are on Phase Two. Or, once you are happy with following the programme, you can choose your lunches and evening meals from the free choices that follow on pages 72–73.
● Read all the instructions on pages 53–60 before beginning, and don't forget your daily allowance of milk and your unlimited items, including up to 8 glasses of water a day.

· *Day One* ·

Breakfast
Choose one from the list on pages 59–60.

Mid-morning snack
Choose one selection from the PHASE TWO BEST MIXES on page 58.

Lunch
1 portion Ham, Egg and Potato Salad (see recipe, page 105) plus 1 medium slice dark rye bread.

Mid-afternoon snack
As morning.

Evening Meal
1 portion Penne with Tuna and Olives (see recipe, page 85) with a mixed salad.

For vegetarians: Use 100g (3¹/₂ oz) mushrooms per person instead of the tuna.

· *Day Two* ·

Breakfast
Choose from the list on pages 59–60.

Mid-morning snack
As Day One.

Lunch

1 portion Pasta and Bean Soup (see recipe page 81) with medium slice dark rye bread; 1 banana.

or

300 ml (1/2 pint) fresh ready-made minestrone soup.

Mid-afternoon snack

As Day One.

Evening Meal

1 portion Chilli Chicken (see recipe, page 96) with 25g (1oz) dry weight noodles or brown rice, cooked, plus two or three portions fresh vegetables, e.g., cabbage, broccoli or spinach.

   For vegetarians: Use Quorn or TVP chunks in the recipe instead of the chicken and vegetable stock.

· *Day Three* ·

Breakfast

Choose one from the list on pages 59–60.

Mid-morning snack

As Day One.

Lunch

Sandwich of 2 medium slices dark rye bread with a little low-fat spread filled with 100g (31/2oz) tuna in brine, drained, and unlimited salad

or

5 medium sardines, grilled, with 1 wholemeal pitta bread or large slice rye bread and large mixed salad. 1 banana with either choice.

Mid-afternoon snack

As Day One.

Evening Meal

1 portion Mushroom Risotto (see recipe, page 99), 1 diet yogurt, 1 plum or apricot or 25g (1oz) cherries.

· *Day Four* ·

Breakfast
Choose one from the list on pages 59–60.

Mid-morning snack
As Day One.

Lunch
1 portion Cheese, Pineapple and Pasta Salad (see recipe, page 106)

Mid-afternoon snack
As Day One.

Evening
1 x 110g (4oz) salmon steak or fillet, baked in foil and served with 110g (4oz) cooked weight green lentils, one portion fresh green vegetable; 1 apple.

For vegetarians: Mix the lentils with some Italian tomato sauce and serve with 200g (7oz) cooked weight couscous or bulgar wheat and 1 tablespoon grated cheese on top.

· *Day Five* ·

Breakfast
Choose one from the list on pages 59–60.

Mid-morning snack
As Day One.

Lunch
1 portion Lentil Soup (see recipe, page 80) plus 1 medium slice dark rye bread; 1 apple.

Mid-afternoon snack
As Day One.

Evening
1 portion Ratatouille and Eggs in a Baked Herb Crust (see recipe, page 100) with 50g (2oz) dark rye bread and a little low-fat spread; 1 orange or peach.

· *Day Six* ·

Breakfast
Choose one from the list on pages 59–60.

Mid-morning snack
As Day One.

Lunch
200g (7oz) baked beans or curried beans on 50g (2oz) rye bread, toasted; 1 apple.

Mid-afternoon snack
As Day One.

Evening
Stir fry: 100g (3$^{1}/_2$ oz) extra lean beef or pork, cut into strips and stir fried with 225g (8oz) mixed fresh vegetables of choice plus 2 tablespoons hoisin sauce, using 1 dessertspoon corn oil in the wok. Serve with 50g (2oz) dry weight egg thread noodles, cooked according to packet instructions.

*For vegetarians: Use 25g (1oz) flaked almonds *or* 100g (3$^{1}/_2$ oz) tofu chunks instead of the meat.

· *Day Seven* ·

Breakfast
Choose one from the list on pages 59–60.

Mid-morning snack
As Day One.

Lunch
1 wholemeal pitta bread filled with 100g (3$^{1}/_2$ oz) canned or fresh, cooked, flaked salmon plus 2 tablespoons 8% fat fromage frais blended with 1 level teaspoon French mustard, and chopped spring onions, red pepper, lettuce and cucumber.

*For vegetarians: Use 40g (1$^{1}/_2$ oz) cubed Edam or 50g (2oz) cubed Feta cheese instead of the salmon.

Mid-afternoon snack
As Day One.

Evening
1 portion Gratin of Pulses and Vegetables (see recipe, page 101) served with 50g (2oz) dry weight barley, couscous or bulgar wheat, cooked or soaked according to packet instructions.

· *Phase Two Freechoice Lunches* ·

Vary your choices as much as possible.

- Any lunch from the Phase Two set diet.
- Any lunch from the Phase One set diet.
- 1 size 3 egg, poached or boiled, with 2 tomatoes, grilled, 1 low-fat pork chipolata, grilled, 50g (2oz) dark rye bread; 1 apple.
- 75g (3oz) hummus with 3 dark rye Ryvitas, large mixed salad; 1 orange or peach; 1 diet yogurt.
- Coleslaw made from shredded white cabbage, grated carrot and onion with 1 tablespoon sultanas, dressed with 1 tablespoon each of low-fat natural Bio yogurt and 70% fat-free mayonnaise, blended. Serve with 50g (2oz) extra lean ham or cottage cheese plus 50g (2oz) dark rye bread; 2 plums or apricots.
- 6 tablespoons cooked couscous mixed with a selection of chopped salad vegetables plus 50g (2oz) lean cooked chicken, chopped, and oil-free French dressing, served with 2 Ryvitas; 1 diet yogurt; 1 small banana.
- Salad of 100g (3¹/2 oz) cooked butterbeans mixed with 100g (3¹/2 oz) flaked tuna in brine, drained, 1 large tomato, chopped, 4 black olives, stoned, and 4 spring onions, chopped. Serve on salad leaves with 1 medium slice dark rye bread. Toss the salad in oil-free French dressing.
- 1 x 550ml (1 pint) carton fresh (chilled counter) onion soup topped with 2 tablespoons grated Parmesan cheese and served with 50g (2oz) dark rye bread.
- 200g (7oz) cooked weight pasta spirals tossed with oil-free French dressing plus a selection of chopped mixed vegetables, 25g (1oz) sultanas, 25g (1oz) Edam cheese and 1 piece fruit of choice.
- 2 savoury oatcakes with 1 small tub cottage cheese, celery and tomato salad, followed by 1 breakfast muffin and 1 apple.
- 1 x 100g (3¹/2 oz) VegeBurger inside 1 wholegrain bap; large mixed salad; 1 peach, 1 diet yogurt.
- 150g (5oz) mixed canned beans, tossed with 4 tablespoons Italian tomato sauce and 200g (7oz) cooked weight pasta spirals or shells plus sliced mushrooms.
- 2 large open-cup mushrooms de-stalked and filled with 1 portion Spicy Rice Stuffing (see recipe, page 109) drizzled with vegetable stock and covered in foil, baked for 20 minutes or until piping hot; 1 apple, 1 diet fromage frais.

· *Phase Two Freechoice* · Evening Meals

- Any evening meal from the Phase Two set diet.
- 1 portion Sesame Prawns (see recipe, page 92 with 50g (2oz) dry weight egg thread noodles, cooked according to packet instructions, plus green side salad.
- 1 portion Seared Tuna Steaks with Warm Piquant Dressing (see recipe, page 93); 200g (7oz) boiled potatoes; 2 servings fresh vegetables of choice.
- 1 portion Spicy Rice Stuffing (see recipe, page 109) with 125g (4$^{1}/_{2}$ oz) lean chicken meat, cooked, mixed in and heated; large mixed salad.
- 1 small rainbow trout, cooked without added fat (e.g., steamed, grilled or microwaved); 200g (7oz) new potatoes, one portion peas, one portion broccoli.
- 1 portion Lamb and Lentil Casserole (see recipe, page 97) served with 6 tablespoons cooked couscous and 1 green vegetable of choice.
- 1 large sweet potato, baked and topped with 2 tablespoons 8% fat fromage frais beaten with 1 level teaspoon mild curry powder; 1 well grilled bacon rasher chopped; large mixed salad with oil-free French dressing.
- 2 falafel (chick pea) patties (from chilled or frozen counter), cooked in a non-stick frying pan with a little Fry Light spray; 1 200g (7oz) portion cooked brown rice; 3 tablespoons spicy tomato sauce (from jar); 2 servings green vegetables.
- 1 x 125g (4$^{1}/_{2}$ oz) turkey steak, grilled; 1 small sweet potato, peeled, cubed and boiled then mashed with 1 teaspoon olive oil and seasoning; 2 portions vegetables of choice.
- 2-egg omelette cooked in non-stick pan with a little Fry Light spray and filled with 50g (2oz) mushrooms; 50g (2oz) dark rye bread; large mixed salad with oil-free French dressing.
- 1 large cod or other white fish fillet, baked in foil or microwaved in parchment with lemon juice, seasoning, chives or dill, and julienne strips of carrot and courgette; served with 175g (6oz) boiled potato; 2 portions vegetables of choice and 1 tablespoon grated Cheddar cheese.

· *PHASE THREE* ·

The seven-day set diet

- The seven days can be repeated if necessary, although for most women, they should easily cover any Phase Three phase, after which you will return to Phase One in a normal cycle, or perhaps Phase Two, if you are following a different routine (say, if you don't have periods).
- Read all the instructions on pages 53–60 before beginning, and don't forget your daily allowance of milk and your unlimited items, including up to 8 glasses of water a day.

· *Day One* ·

Breakfast
Choose one from the list on pages 59–60.

Mid-morning snack
Choose one selection from the PHASE THREE BEST MIXES on page 58.

Lunch
225g (8oz) low-sugar, low-salt baked beans in tomato sauce on 50g (2oz) slice dark rye toast with a little low-fat spread; 1 satsuma; 1 apple
or
have 100g (3¹/₂ oz) butter bean purée PLUS the bread and fruit, followed by a diet yogurt.

Mid-afternoon snack
As morning.

Evening
1 portion Vegetable and Pasta Gratin (see recipe, page 86), 1 banana.

· *Day Two* ·

Breakfast
Choose one from the list on pages 59–60.

Mid-morning snack
As Day One.

Lunch
1 wholemeal pitta bread filled with 40g (1½ oz) Edam cheese, chopped, and mixed with 1 level dessertspoon 70% fat-free mayonnaise, a selection of mixed chopped salad vegetables and 20g chopped mixed nuts.

Mid-afternoon snack
As Day One.

Evening
1 portion Beany Cottage Pie (see recipe, page 98) served with a portion of sweetcorn or peas and a leafy green vegetable of choice; 1 apple; 1 diet fromage frais.

· *Day Three* ·

Breakfast
Choose one from the list on pages 59–60.

Mid-morning snack
As Day One.

Lunch
1 portion Mixed Bean Salad with Fruit (see recipe, page 106); 1 apple.

Mid-afternoon snack
As Day One.

Evening
1 portion Buckwheat Pancakes with Mushrooms and Cheese Sauce (see recipe, page 101), large mixed salad with oil-free French dressing; 1 orange.

· *Day Four* ·

Breakfast
Choose one from the list on pages 59–60.

Mid-morning snack
As Day One.

Lunch
75g (3oz) hummus with 1 wholemeal pitta bread, mixed salad, 1 plum or apricot, 50g (2oz) cherries.

Mid-afternoon snack
As Day One.

Evening
1 portion Seafood Lasagne (see recipe, page 87) plus a large mixed salad with oil-free French dressing
   For vegetarians: 1 portion Tagliatelle with a Mixed Vegetable Sauce (see recipe, page 84) plus 1 banana.

· *Day Five* ·

Breakfast
Choose one from the list on pages 59–60.

Mid-morning snack
As Day One.

Lunch
1 portion Provençal Salad with Goat's Cheese (see recipe, page 107) plus 1 apple.

Mid-afternoon snack
As Day One.

Evening
1 portion Chinese Noodles with Chicken (see recipe, page 88), 1 diet yogurt.
   For vegetarians: Use tofu in the Noodle recipe instead of the chicken.

· *Day Six* ·

Breakfast
Choose one from the list on pages 59–60.

Mid-morning snack
As Day One.

Lunch
Salad: Mix 1 small can tuna in water, drained and flaked, with 100g (3^1/$_2$ oz) cooked flageolet beans, 1 large tomato, chopped, 1 shallot, chopped and 1 hard-boiled egg, sliced. Toss in oil-free French dressing and serve with 1 medium slice dark rye bread; 1 orange.

Mid-afternoon snack
As Day One.

Evening
1 portion Spiced Potato and Aubergine (see recipe, page 103) with 200g (7oz) cooked weight couscous or bulgar wheat; large mixed salad (no dressing).

· *Day Seven* ·

Breakfast
Choose one from the list on pages 59–60.

Mid-morning snack
As Day One.

Lunch
1 portion Lentil Soup (see recipe, page 80 plus 50g (2oz) slice dark rye bread; 1 apple.

Mid-afternoon snack
As Day One.

Evening
1 portion Fettuccine with avocado and bacon (see recipe pages 88); green salad.
   For vegetarians: Substitute 100g (3^1/$_2$ oz) half fat mozzarella cheese for the bacon (per whole, 4-portion recipe).

· *Phase Three Freechoice* · Lunches

Vary your choices as much as possible.

- Any lunch from the Phase Three set diet.
- 1 portion Pasta and Bean Soup (see recipe, page 81) plus 1 pitta bread; 1 small banana.
- 1 portion Potato and Broccoli Soup (see recipe, page 82) with 2 tablespoons Parmesan cheese and 50g (2oz) dark rye bread with a little low-fat spread; 1 apple.
- 1 portion Prawn Salad with Cashews (see recipe, page 108).
- 1 portion Baby Vegetable and Chicken Salad (see recipe, page 104) served with 3 dark rye Ryvitas with a little low-fat spread; 1 piece of fruit of your choice.
- 1 portion Pasta and Tuna Salad (see recipe, page 104); 1 portion of fruit of choice.
- 1 portion Cheese, Pineapple and Pasta Salad (see recipe, page 106); 1 apple.
- 100g (3 1/2 oz) mushrooms, sliced and stir-fried in 1 dessert-spoon olive oil, seasoned, served on 50g (2oz) dark rye toast with 2 tablespoons Parmesan cheese; 1 diet yogurt; 1 banana.
- 275ml (1/2 pint) fresh (chilled counter) vegetable soup of choice (not 'cream of. . .'), e.g., spinach and nutmeg or carrot and tomato; 3 savoury oatcakes; 1 small tub cottage cheese, mixed salad with oil-free French dressing; 1 slice canteloupe melon or 3 fresh apricots.
- Open sandwiches – 2 medium slices dark rye bread spread with a little medium-fat goat's cheese; one topped with 1 tablespoon chopped nuts, chopped apple and celery; the other topped with 1 dessertspoon pine nuts, chopped dried apricot and cucumber; 2 plums.

· *Phase Three Freechoice* ·
Evening Meals

- Any evening meal from the Phase Three set diet.
- 1 portion Chicken and Pistachio Pilau (see recipe, page 95).
- 1 portion Chicken Tuscany (see recipe, page 97) served with 50g (2oz) dry weight pasta of choice, boiled; plus 1 serving of green vegetable of choice.
- 1 portion Chilli Chicken (see recipe, page 96) served with 200g (7oz) cooked weight couscous or bulgar wheat; salad.
- 1 portion Turkey and Nut Stir Fry (see recipe, page 94) served with 40g (1$^{1}/_2$ oz) dry weight egg thread noodles, cooked according to packet instructions.
- 1 medium portion roast chicken ($^{1}/_4$ of a small chicken) without skin, with 1 medium sweet potato, baked, and 2 portions green vegetables; 1 peach or nectarine.
- 1 portion Ratatouille and Eggs in a Baked Herb Crust (see recipe, page 100); 50g (2oz) dark rye bread; 1 apple.
- 1 x 110g (4oz) salmon fillet or steak, cooked without added fat (e.g., grilled or microwaved); served with a sauce of 2 tablespoons 8% fat fromage frais mixed with 1 teaspoon Dijon wholegrain mustard; 175g (6oz) cooked weight brown rice; 1 portion broccoli, 1 portion peas.
- 75g (3oz) dry weight pasta ribbons, cooked and topped with 3 tablespoons ready-made pesto mixed with 1 large tomato, de-seeded and chopped; green salad.
- 1 portion Lamb and Lentil Casserole (see recipe, page 97) with 1 small sweet potato, baked, plus 1 leafy green vegetable.

5

THE BODYSENSE RECIPES

· SOUPS AND SNACKS ·

· Lentil Soup ·

Serves 4
290 calories; 6g fat per portion

1 tablespoon olive oil
1 large onion, finely chopped
325g (12oz) brown or green lentils,
    washed
1 litre (1³/4 pints) vegetable or
    chicken stock
2 stalks celery, chopped

1 large carrot, chopped
3 canned tomatoes, drained and
    roughly chopped
1 clove garlic, crushed
A little salt
Black pepper

Heat the oil in a large saucepan over medium heat and add onions; sauté, stirring occasionally, until soft. Add the lentils and stir for a minute, then add the rest of the ingredients. Lower heat to simmer, put the lid on the pan, and simmer for about an hour, or until the lentils are tender. Check seasoning.

TIPS
- You can purée all the soup in a blender for a thick, creamy texture (and the soup will be easier to digest). Or you could purée half of it so you have a thick texture but also some 'bite' left.
- You must use brown or green lentils for this recipe; the orange ones aren't as tasty.
- You can use split peas instead of lentils; and you can add a little lean cooked ham too, if you like, which will add around 40 calories and 1.5g fat per 25g (1oz). Add the ham, cut into small chunks, when the soup is cooked and after puréeing.

· *Pasta and Bean Soup* ·

Serves 4
195 calories; 6g fat per portion

1 large stalk celery
1 medium courgette
1 medium leek
75g (3oz) white cabbage
1 medium carrot
1 large onion
75g (3oz) broccoli
1 clove garlic, crushed
1 tablespoon olive oil
200g (7oz) can chopped tomatoes

825ml (1^1/$_2$ pints) chicken stock
100g (3^1/$_2$ oz) dry weight small
pasta shapes
1 x 200g (7oz) can butterbeans,
drained
1 tablespoon tomato purée
A little salt
Black pepper
1 tablespoon chopped parsley
1 tablespoon grated Parmesan

Chop all the vegetables except the broccoli finely. Cut the broccoli into very small florets. Heat the oil in a large saucepan, add all the vegetables except the broccoli, and add the garlic. Stir for 3 minutes over a medium heat. Add the tomatoes, stock and pasta, stir and simmer for 30 minutes. Add the butterbeans, tomato purée, seasoning and broccoli and simmer for 10 minutes. Check seasoning, and serve with the parsley and Parmesan.

TIPS
● Try to buy fresh chicken stock from the chilled counter at the supermarket as it contains less salt than cubes or stock pastes. Or make your own – simmer chicken carcass with carrots and onion, and some parsley for 1 hour or so; sieve and reduce the stock by boiling for a few minutes. Allow to cool then skim any fat that has come to the top before using. (Don't use chicken skin in this stock recipe.)
● Flageolet beans can be used instead of the butterbeans.

· *Potato and Broccoli Soup* ·

Serves 4
165 calories; 2.5g fat per portion

450g (1lb) old potatoes
325g (12oz) broccoli head
700ml (1¼ pints) chicken stock
275ml (½ pint) semi-skimmed
 milk

1 small onion, finely chopped
A little salt
Black pepper

Peel the potatoes and cut them into small chunks. Remove any leaves and very tough stalk from the broccoli and cut into small florets. Put all the ingredients into a large saucepan and simmer for 25 minutes. Pour the soup into a blender and liquidize until smooth and creamy. Pour back into the pan, reheat, check seasoning and serve.

· *Cheese and Onion Dip* ·

Serves 4
70 calories; 5g fat per portion

50ml Kraft 70% fat-free
 mayonnaise
50g Philadelphia Light cheese
100g (3½ oz) 8% fat fromage
 frais

2 spring onions, finely chopped
1 dessertspoon fresh chopped
 chives
Dash Tabasco (chilli sauce)

In a small bowl, beat the mayonnaise and light cheese together. Gradually beat in the fromage frais, then add the onions and chives. Add Tabasco sparingly to taste.

TIPS
- Serve with crudités and rye crispbreads or pitta strips and salad.
- You can omit the Tabasco if you like – add a little tomato purée in its place.
- If you have no fresh chives, add an extra spring onion.

· *Breakfast Muffins* ·

Makes 8
135 calories; 4g fat per muffin

100g (3^1/$_2$ oz) rolled oats
50g (2oz) plain flour
50g (2oz) buckwheat flour
1 heaped tablespoon fructose
1 heaped teaspoon baking powder
^{1}/$_2$ teaspoon ground cinnamon
75ml (3fl oz) apple juice

50ml (2fl oz) skimmed milk
1 egg
1 tablespoon corn oil
1 eating apple
50g (2oz) blackcurrants or berry
  fruit

Heat the oven to 200°C, 400°F, Gas Mark 6. Coat muffin tin bases and sides with cooking oil spray. Combine the dry ingredients, then in another bowl, mix together the apple juice, milk, egg and oil. Core the apple and chop it into small pieces; add apple and currants or berries to the wet mixture, then fold in the dry ingredients. Divide mixture between eight muffin tin moulds and bake for about 18 minutes or until the muffins are risen and golden.

TIPS
● These muffins will freeze.
● Experiment with other fruits in your muffins – fresh apricots or peaches, stoned cherries or plums are all good – and good for you.

· *PASTA DISHES* ·

· *Chicken and Pasta Peperonata* ·

Serves 4
320 calories; 10g fat per serving

4 average chicken breast portions,
  skinned and boned
1 tablespoon plain flour
1^1/$_2$ tablespoons olive oil
1 large red onion, sliced
1 clove garlic, crushed
3 large mixed peppers (about 400g
  or 14oz)

1 x 400g (14oz) can chopped
  tomatoes with herbs
A little salt
Black pepper
8 stoned black olives, halved
200g (7oz) dry weight pappardelle
  pasta
Fresh basil

Cut the chicken into bite-sized strips and toss in the flour. Heat 1 tablespoon of the oil in a large frying pan and sear the chicken until golden. Remove with a slotted spoon on to a plate. Add the rest of the oil and stir-fry the onion, garlic and peppers over a high heat for 3–4 minutes. Add the tomatoes and seasoning and return the chicken to the pan. Turn the heat down and simmer for 20 minutes or until the peppers are soft, adding the olives for the last minute or two.

Meanwhile, cook the pasta in a large pan of boiling, salted water, until *al dente* – about 10 minutes – and drain. Toss the pasta with the chicken sauce and serve with basil leaves to garnish.

TIPS

- Pappardelle is a flat pasta cut into thick ribbons – a little like tagliatelle but wider. If you can't get it, tagliatelle will do.
- This dish will freeze – undercook it slightly before freezing.
- Vegetarians can make the dish using Quorn chunks or chestnut mushrooms – add some grated Parmesan to increase the protein content of the recipe if using mushrooms.

· *Tagliatelle with Mixed Vegetable* · *Sauce*

Serves 4
405 calories; 7g fat per portion

1 tablespoon olive oil
1 small onion, finely chopped
1 large leek, cut into thin rounds
1 small courgette, sliced into thin strips
1 clove garlic, crushed
25g (1oz) sun-dried tomatoes, chopped
4 large tomatoes, skinned and
    chopped
200ml (7fl oz) Passata
1 tablespoon tomato purée

Pinch fructose
Dash Worcestershire sauce
1 teaspoon chopped oregano
A little salt
Black pepper
200g (7oz) small mushrooms
325g (12oz) spinach tagliatelle
50g (2oz) 8% fat fromage frais
4 tablespoons Parmesan cheese

Heat the oil in a large sauté pan; add the onion and leek, and stir for 3 minutes over a medium to high heat. Add the courgette and garlic, and stir for two minutes. Add the sun-dried tomatoes, chopped tomatoes and Passata, tomato purée, fructose, Worcester-shire sauce and seasoning, and simmer, covered, for 10 minutes. Add the mushrooms and simmer for another 10 minutes or until the sauce is rich (add a little extra Passata if it looks too dry).

Meanwhile, cook the tagliatelle in a large pan of boiling, salted water until *al dente*. When the pasta and sauce are ready, stir the fromage frais into the sauce and check seasoning. Toss with the pasta and serve topped with the cheese.

TIPS
- Use aubergine instead of the mushrooms for a change. Bake an aubergine in its skin (prick first) then scoop out the flesh.
- You could use a can of chopped tomatoes if you are in a hurry, instead of the fresh tomatoes and Passata.

· *Penne with Tuna and Olives* ·

Serves 4
480 calories; 12g fat per portion

$1/2$ tablespoon olive oil
Level tablespoon butter
4 small tuna steaks (100g or $3^1/2$ oz each)
1 onion, finely chopped
2 cloves garlic, crushed
2 tomatoes, skinned and chopped
A little salt

Black pepper
1 teaspoon chopped thyme
1 glass (140ml) dry white wine
3 tablespoons chopped, flat-leaved parsley
12 black olives; stoned and halved
275g (10oz) penne pasta, dry weight

Heat the oil and butter in a large sauté pan and sear the tuna steaks over a high heat, 1 minute on both sides. Remove with a slatted spoon, add the onion and garlic and stir-fry over a medium heat for 5 minutes or until the onion is soft. Add the rest of the ingredients except the pasta, parsley and olives to the pan and simmer for 15 minutes until sauce is rich. Flake the tuna and add to the sauce; simmer for 3–4 minutes. Stir the parsley and olives in.

Meanwhile, cook the pasta in a large pan of boiling salted water until *al dente*. Serve the pasta drained and tossed with the sauce.

TIPS

- You can use canned tuna if you like; drain it well; don't sear but just add after the sauce is made.
- Fresh mussels work well in this dish instead of the tuna. Omit the olives and add an extra tomato. To cook, add the mussels and white wine to the pan when the onions are soft, cover and steam for 5 minutes until the mussels are open. (Remember to discard any muscles that do not open.) Then proceed as above.

· *Vegetable and Pasta Gratin* ·

Serves 4
430 calories; 13g fat per portion

1 large aubergine, cut into chunks
2 medium red onions, cut into chunks
1 red pepper, de-seeded and cut into squares
4 small courgettes, cut into chunks
200g (7oz) dry weight macaroni
1 quantity cheese sauce (see recipe, page 110)

150g (5^1/$_2$ oz) broccoli
50g (2oz) sun-dried tomatoes, chopped
1 tablespoon olive oil
25g (1oz) dry breadcrumbs
1 teaspoon mixed Mediterranean herbs
A little salt
Black pepper

Toss the aubergine, onion, pepper and courgettes in the oil and spread on a baking tray. Season lightly. Roast at 200°C, 400°F, Gas Mark 6 for 40 minutes, or until tender and golden, turning once. Meanwhile, parboil the broccoli in a little water, drain and reserve. Cook the pasta in a large pan of boiling, salted water, drain and reserve. Make the cheese sauce if you haven't already done so.

In a family-sized gratin dish, arrange the roasted vegetables with the broccoli, sun-dried tomatoes and pasta, plus any juices from the roasting pan. Top with the cheese sauce, then sprinkle over the breadcrumbs, herbs and seasoning. Return to the oven and bake until the top is golden – about 20 minutes.

TIP

- Don't buy sun-dried tomatoes in oil, but the ones that come in a vacuum pack. They are much lower in calories.

· *Seafood Lasagne* ·

Serves 4
430 calories; 10g fat per portion

1 tablespoon olive oil
1 leek
1 x 400g (14oz) can chopped
 tomatoes
1 tablespoon tomato purée
A little fish stock
450g (1lb) white fish fillet
100g (3^1/2 oz) sliced mushrooms

1 dessertspoon fresh chopped basil,
 or 1 teaspoon dried
325g (12oz) peeled prawns
8 lasagne sheets, 'no need to pre-
 cook' variety
75g (3oz) half-fat grated Mozzarella
A little salt
Black pepper

Preheat the oven to 180°C, 350°F, Gas Mark 4. Heat the oil in a large sauté pan and stir-fry the leek for 3 minutes over a medium heat. Add the tomatoes, tomato purée, and a little fish stock. Simmer for 15 minutes. Cut the fish into chunks and add it to the pan with the prawns and mushrooms. Simmer for 5 minutes. Add the basil, stir and remove from heat.

Spread a third of the fish mixture over the base of a square lasagne dish and cover with four of the lasagne sheets. Spread another third of the mixture over, then arrange the remaining lasagne sheets. Finish with the remainder of the mixture and sprinkle the cheese over the top. Bake for 30 minutes or until the cheese has turned golden.

TIPS

- When using 'no pre-cook' lasagne, the sauce mixture needs to be fairly liquid, as the pasta needs to absorb the liquid while the dish is baking. So, if the sauce is anything drier than a thick soup, add extra fish stock to it before spreading in the dish.
- For an inexpensive dish you can omit the prawns and use extra white fish. You can, of course, use other seafood, too, such as mussels or crab sticks.

· *Chinese Noodles with Chicken* ·

Serves 4
465 calories; 8g fat per portion

300g (11oz) medium egg thread
    noodles
1 carrot
1 large stick celery
1 green pepper, de-seeded
50g (2oz) mangetout or green beans
6 spring onions
100g (3½ oz) mushrooms

1 tablespoon groundnut or sesame
    oil
325g (12oz) lean chicken meat,
    chopped
1–2 tablespoons soya sauce
275ml (½ pint) chicken stock
1 level dessertspoon cornflour
2 slices pineapple, chopped

Boil the noodles in water for 4 minutes or as instructed on the packet, drain and leave, covered.

Slice all the vegetables thinly into even pieces; heat the oil in a wok or large non-stick frying pan and stir-fry the vegetables and the chicken for 3 minutes. Add soya sauce to taste, a little of the chicken stock, and stir-fry again for another 3 minutes. When the vegetables are cooked but still firm, mix the remaining chicken stock with the cornflour and add to pan with the pineapple. Stir until sauce has thickened. Add noodles to wok, stir to heat through and serve.

TIP

● You can use a variety of different vegetables in this dish, to replace some or all of those listed above – for example, broccoli, peas, leeks, courgette.

· *Fettuccine with Avocado and Bacon* ·

Serves 4
475 calories; 16g fat per portion

325g (12oz) dry weight fettuccine
4 thin rashers extra-lean, low-salt
    back bacon, chopped
4 large shallots, chopped finely
2 medium avocados
1 tablespoon lemon juice

150ml (5½ fl oz) 8% fat fromage
    frais
A little salt
Black pepper
2 tablespoons chopped parsley
4 tablespoons Parmesan cheese

Cook the pasta in a large pan of boiling, salted water until *al dente*. Meanwhile, put the bacon in a heavy, non-stick frying pan over a low heat and gradually increase the heat as the bacon cooks in its own fat (even low-fat bacon will do this). When the bacon is beginning to crisp, add the shallots and stir for a few minutes. Peel and stone the avocados and mash with the lemon juice. Add to the pan with the fromage frais, and stir over a low heat until you have a smooth sauce. Season to taste. Drain the pasta and toss with the sauce. Serve garnished with the parsley and Parmesan.

TIPS

- Have a large mixed salad with this pasta dish.
- The dish sounds over-indulgent but in fact much of the fat content is unsaturated – and avocados are a good source of vitamin E.

· *FISH AND SEAFOOD* ·

· *Baked Salmon and Rice with a* · *Creamed Coulis*

Serves 4
380 calories; 15g fat per portion

200g (7oz) dry weight brown rice	A little salt
100g (3^1/$_2$ oz) fresh broccoli	Black pepper
4 x 100g (3^1/$_2$ oz) salmon steaks	2 tablespoons low-fat crème
50ml (2fl oz) fish stock	fraîche

Boil the brown rice in lightly salted water in a covered pan until soft but retaining a little 'bite'. Meanwhile, steam the broccoli and grill, bake, microwave or steam the salmon steaks until just cooked. When the broccoli is cooked, purée it in a blender with the fish stock. Season to taste and stir in the crème fraîche. Serve the salmon with the broccoli coulis and the rice.

TIPS

- Take care not to overcook the salmon or it will dry out.
- Serve with mangetout or peas or green beans.
- A red pepper sauce also goes well – de-seed, quarter, grill until charred and skin a large red pepper and proceed as above using it instead of the broccoli.

· *Salmon and Spinach Pie* ·

Serves 4
360 calories; 15g fat per portion

100g (3^1/$_2$ oz) mixed white and
   wild rice
250g (9oz) salmon fillet
100g (3^1/$_2$ oz) smoked haddock
   fillet
2 size 3 eggs
6 spring onions, chopped
100g (3^1/$_2$ oz) button mushrooms,
   sliced

Juice of 1 lime
2 tablespoons chopped parsley
2 tablespoons grated Parmesan
200ml (7fl oz) half-fat Greek yogurt
Pinch paprika
A little salt
Black pepper
1 x 250g (9oz) packet leaf spinach,
   thawed if frozen.

Cook the rice in lightly salted boiling water as instructed on
packet. Poach, steam or microwave the fish until barely cooked
and flake it. Boil the eggs until hard. Now simply mix all the
ingredients except the spinach together and place in a lightly oiled
baking dish. If using fresh spinach, wilt it lightly in a saucepan.
Arrange the spinach over the top of the fish mixture evenly, cover
with foil or a lid and bake at 180°C, 350°F, Gas Mark 4 for 25
minutes before serving.

TIPS
● You can use tuna instead of the salmon in this dish.
● You can use frozen spinach for the topping but it has to be
   whole leaf spinach, not chopped.

· *Grilled Cod with a Tomato and* ·
Red Pepper Salsa

Serves 4
190 calories; 2.5g fat per portion

4 large tomatoes, skinned, de-seeded
   and chopped
8 black stoned olives, chopped
1 red onion, chopped
1 medium red pepper, skinned and
   chopped
1 tablespoon fresh coriander, chopped

Juice of 2 limes
A little salt
Black pepper
Dash Tabasco
4 medium cod fillets
Lime wedges

Combine the first nine ingredients in a bowl, cover and leave in the fridge for several hours if possible. Grill the cod fillets and serve the cod with the salsa and lime wedges.

TIPS

- To skin red pepper, de-seed it and cut into four, then place under a hot grill until the skin begins to blacken. Leave to cool slightly then slip the skin off with your fingers. As a quicker alternative, you can buy cans of ready skinned red 'piquillo' peppers, though they are quite expensive.
- You can substitute halibut, swordfish or fresh tuna for the cod in this recipe.

· *Quick Sautéed Fish and Tomato* · *Sauce*

Serves 4
200 calories; 2.5g fat per portion

4 shallots or 1 mild sweet onion, finely chopped	1 heaped tablespoon 70% fat-free mayonnaise
4 medium tomatoes, skinned and de-seeded	1 level tablespoon French mustard
5 tablespoons fish stock	4 medium white fish fillets, e.g., cod
A little salt	1 tablespoon wholemeal flour, seasoned
Black pepper	Fry Light cooking spray

In a small saucepan, simmer the shallots, tomatoes, stock and seasoning for 30 minutes and then put through a blender (or through a sieve). Return to the pan and keep warm.

Mix the mayonnaise and mustard, and use to coat the fish fillets, then dip the fillets in the flour. Heat a large heavy-based frying pan with the Fry Light and gently sauté the fish, turning once. Sauté for 10–15 minutes, depending upon the thickness of your fish. Serve with the sauce.

TIP

- To prepare tomatoes, make a cross across the top and blanch them in boiling water for 1 minute. Peel off skins; halve the tomatoes and gently press out the seeds.

· *Tuna Fish Cakes* ·

Serves 4
250 calories; 6g fat per portion

1 x 400g (14oz) can tuna in brine, drained
400g (14oz) mashed potato
150ml (5¹/2 fl oz) skimmed milk
1 small onion, finely chopped
2 tablespoons chopped parsley

1 tablespoon reduced-fat mayonnaise (e.g., Hellmann's)
1 size 3 egg
A little salt
Black pepper
1 dessertspoon corn oil

In a bowl, mix all the ingredients except the oil. Form into 8 patties and place on a baking sheet brushed with the corn oil. Bake for 20 minutes or so, turning once, or until the cakes are golden.

TIPS

- You can make fresh mashed potato (using skimmed milk to mash, and no butter) or you can use a good-quality instant mash.
- Try other fish in this recipe, such as salmon or smoked cod.
- The cakes are good with the tomato sauce in the previous recipe.

· *Sesame Prawns* ·

Serves 4
225 calories; 11g fat per portion

2 tablespoons sesame oil
8 large spring onions, each cut into quarters lengthways
1 large red pepper, de-seeded and cut into strips
1 clove garlic, finely chopped
450g (1lb) uncooked large prawns
1 small red chilli, de-seeded and finely chopped

1 tablespoon rich soya sauce
Pinch sugar
1 tablespoon sesame seeds
Juice of 1 lime
2 tablespoons fresh chopped coriander or parsley
Black pepper

Heat half the oil in a wok and stir-fry the onion and red pepper on high for 2–3 minutes. Add the chilli, garlic and prawns, fry and stir for another 2 minutes. Add the rest of the ingredients and stir for a minute. Drizzle the remaining oil over the dish before serving.

TIPS

● Serve with Thai fragrant rice, Basmati rice, saffron rice or noodles.
● When handling fresh chillies, don't put your hands near your face or eyes as the chilli will sting you, and wash your hands immediately you have finished preparing the chilli.

· *Seared Tuna Steaks with Warm* · *Piquant Dressing*

Serves 4
210 calories; 10g fat per portion

2 tablespoons olive oil
1 tablespoon white wine vinegar
1 tablespoon drained capers
1 tomato, skinned, de-seeded and chopped
1 clove garlic, very finely chopped (optional)

1 tablespoon chopped parsley
A little salt
Black pepper
4 x 100g (3½ oz) tuna steaks
Fry Light spray

Combine the first eight ingredients very well (in a screw top jar if you have one). Heat a large, heavy-based sauté pan sprayed with Fry Light until very hot and sear the tuna on each side for 2 minutes; turn the heat down and cook for a further 2 minutes (or longer) to taste. Remove the steaks from the pan and keep warm. Add the dressing to the pan, stir and allow to bubble, then immediately remove from the heat and pour over the steaks.

TIPS

● You can blend the dressing in a blender if you like but you will get a different result; I prefer the sauce unblended but very thoroughly mixed.
● Tuna can be dry if overcooked so watch your steaks – if necessary, cut a sneaky slit in one (yours!) to see if it is sufficiently cooked. Still slightly pink in the centre is about right.

· *POULTRY AND MEAT* ·

· *Turkey and Nut Stir Fry* ·

Serves 4
332 calories; 19g fat per portion

100ml (3½ fl oz) pineapple juice
1 tablespoon hoisin sauce
1 tablespoon plum sauce
1 tablespoon soya sauce
1 dessertspoon cornflour
1 teaspoon ground ginger
1 tablespoon groundnut or corn oil
1 large red pepper, de-seeded and sliced

200g (7oz) broccoli, cut into small florets
100g (3½ oz) mangetout
325g (12oz) turkey fillet, cut into strips
4 shallots, sliced
100g (3 ½ oz) packet toasted flaked almonds

Mix the first six ingredients together in a bowl for a sauce and set aside.

Heat the oil in a wok and stir-fry the red pepper, broccoli and mangetout for 2 minutes on high. Add the turkey and shallots and stir for 3 minutes more. Turn the heat down a little and add the pineapple sauce and the almonds, stir to combine well and cook for 2 minutes before serving.

TIPS

- Vegetarians can substitute tofu chunks or Quorn for the turkey.
- The fat content of this dish seems high but when served with noodles the overall fat content of the dish goes down – also the fat is almost all the 'good for you', unsaturated kind. The highest source of fat in this dish, the almonds, are a super source of vitamin E.

· *Chicken and Pistachio Pilau* ·

Serves 4
500 calories; 14.5g fat per portion

4 chicken breast portions, boneless, skinned
1 tablespoon corn oil
1 medium onion, finely chopped
200g (7oz) long-grain rice
1 teaspoon turmeric
1 teaspoon garam masala
$1/2$ teaspoon cinnamon
A little salt
Black pepper

550ml (1 pint) chicken stock
50g (2oz) sultanas
100g ($3^{1}/2$ oz) cooked chick peas
50g (2oz) shelled pistachio nuts
100ml ($3^{1}/2$ fl oz) natural low-fat yogurt
1 large tomato, skinned, de-seeded and chopped
2 tablespoons chopped coriander leaf

Cut the chicken into small chunks, heat the oil in a large non-stick sauté pan and brown the pieces, removing them to a plate as they turn golden. Stir-fry the onion for 3 minutes then add the rice, spices and seasoning and stir for a few seconds. Add the stock, sultanas and chick peas and return the chicken to the pan. Stir and simmer, covered, for 20 minutes. Add the nuts, yogurt and tomato – and a little extra stock or water if the pilau looks too dry – and simmer again for 2 minutes. Check that the rice is tender (if not, add more stock or water as necessary and simmer again), stir in the coriander and serve.

TIP
● I use canned, drained chick peas for this recipe – you can freeze the surplus for another time.

· *Chilli Chicken* ·

Serves 4
285 calories; 9g fat per portion

4 chicken breast fillets, boneless,
    skinned
1 level tablespoon seasoned flour
1 tablespoon corn oil
2 medium onions, chopped
1 green pepper, de-seeded and
    chopped
1 tablespoon sweet paprika
1 fresh red chilli, de-seeded and
    chopped

250ml ($1/2$ pint) chicken stock
1 x 400g (14oz) can chopped
    tomatoes
A little salt
Black pepper
200g (7oz) cooked red kidney beans
4 tablespoons low-fat Greek yogurt
2 tablespoons chopped parsley

Coat the chicken with the flour, seasoned with a little salt and pepper. Heat the oil in a non-stick lidded sauté pan or flameproof casserole and brown the chicken pieces. Remove from the pan. Add the onion and peppers to the pan and stir-fry for a few minutes, then add the paprika and chilli and stir for another minute, adding a little stock if necessary. Add the rest of the ingredients except the yogurt, parsley and reserved chicken. Simmer, covered, for 30 minutes, then return the chicken to the pan and simmer for another 15 minutes. Check seasoning; stir in the yogurt to serve and garnish with the parsley.

TIP
● Fresh chillies vary a great deal in their heat – often, red ones are hotter than green, and small ones are hotter than large ones. Adjust the amount of chilli you use to take account of this, and your own tastebuds.

· *Chicken Tuscany* ·

Serves 4
250 calories; 9g fat per portion

8 skinless boneless chicken thigh fillets
1 tablespoon seasoned flour
1 tablespoon olive oil
150ml (5fl oz) dry white wine
150ml (5fl oz) chicken stock
150ml (5fl oz) Passata
1 tablespoon tomato purée

1 teaspoon each dried rosemary and thyme
250g (9oz) mushrooms, sliced
A little salt
Black pepper
2 tablespoons half-fat cream

Toss the chicken pieces in seasoned flour. Heat the oil in a flameproof casserole and brown the pieces. Add the rest of the ingredients except the cream, stir, and simmer for 45 minutes, covered *or* cook in the oven at 160°C, 325°F, Gas Mark 3½ until the chicken is tender – about 45 minutes. Stir in the cream before serving.

TIPS
● You can use fresh rosemary and thyme if you have it – a couple a small sprigs of rosemary and four or five of thyme.
● Check the seasoning before adding extra salt or pepper – the seasoned flour may be enough.

· *Lamb and Lentil Casserole* ·

Serves 4
340 calories; 11g fat per portion

Fry Light spray
1 lamb neck fillet, lean trimmed, about 250g (9oz)
150g (5½ oz) brown lentils, dry weight
1 x 400g (14oz) can chopped tomatoes
300ml (11fl oz) lamb, beef or vegetable stock

2 medium onions, chopped
4 medium carrots, cubed
2 large sticks celery, chopped
2 bay leaves
1 teaspoon rosemary
A little salt
Black pepper

Spray a flameproof casserole with Fry Light and brown the lamb pieces, gradually increasing the heat. Add the rest of the ingredients to the pan, stir, cover and simmer for 1¹/2 hours or cook in the oven at 160°C, 325°F, Gas Mark 3¹/2 until the lentils and vegetables are tender. Check halfway through cooking, adding a little more stock if necessary. Check seasoning and serve.

TIP

- Vegetarians can use 100g (4oz) extra lentils, plus 150g (5oz) red kidney beans instead of the lamb, which will make the dish 300 calories and 3g fat per serving.

· *Beany Cottage Pie* ·

1 x 250g (9oz) sweet potato (orange-fleshed kind)
1 x 250g (9oz) baking potato
40ml (1¹/2 fl oz) skimmed milk
250g (9oz) leftover roast lamb leg, finely chopped
1 x 205g (7oz) can low-sugar, low-salt baked beans
1 tablespoon tomato purée

1 medium onion, very finely chopped
1 medium carrot, very finely chopped
125ml (4¹/2 fl oz) strong lamb stock
1 teaspoon mixed dried herbs
1 dessertspoon Worcestershire sauce
Black pepper

Prick the skins of the two kinds of potato and bake for 50 minutes (or until cooked) or microwave for about 10 minutes on high. Scoop out the flesh and mash together with the skimmed milk and seasoning, and set aside.

Mix together the rest of the ingredients in a pie dish, top with the potato mixture and bake at 200°C, 400°F, Gas Mark 6 for 30 minutes.

TIPS

- Vegetarians can use soya mince in this recipe.
- Instead of the baked beans, you could use a can of drained, ready-cooked lentils or mixed beans and add some Passata, or water mixed with tomato purée.
- Chop the onion and carrot into very small pieces – a food processor will do this in seconds.

● If you don't want to bake the potatoes, you could peel them, cut them into chunks and boil them, using the same pan for both, before mashing.

· *Pork and Pepper Stir Fry* ·

Serves 4
225 calories; 11g fat per portion

1 tablespoon corn oil
350g (12^1/$_2$ oz) lean pork fillet, cut into strips
3 mixed peppers (e.g., 1 red, 1 green, 1 yellow), de-seeded and cut into strips
8 spring onions, halved lengthways

2 courgettes, cut into thin ribbons
1–2 tablespoons light soya sauce
1 tablespoon oyster sauce
1 tablespoon chilli sauce
1 dessertspoon runny honey
225g (8oz) beansprouts
200ml (7fl oz) chicken stock mixed with 2 teaspoons cornflour

Heat the oil in a wok and stir-fry the pork and peppers for 3 minutes on high. Add the onions and courgettes and stir for 2 minutes. Add the sauces and honey, and stir for a minute, then add the beansprouts and chicken stock mixture, lower heat and stir for 2 minutes.

TIP
● Vegetarians can use Quorn chunks instead of pork.

· *VEGETARIAN MEALS* ·

· *Mushroom Risotto* ·

Serves 4
400 calories; 13g fat per portion

1^1/$_2$ tablespoons olive oil
1 red onion, finely chopped
300g (11oz) risotto rice, e.g., Arborio
140ml (1 glass) red wine
700ml (1^1/$_2$ pints) vegetable stock
500g (1lb 2oz) mixed mushrooms, sliced as necessary

A little salt
Black pepper
1 tablespoon pine nuts
4 tablespoons Parmesan cheese
2 tablespoons fresh chopped basil

Heat the oil in a large sauté pan and stir the onion for 3 minutes. Add the rice and stir well. Add the wine; bubble, then reduce heat and simmer for 2 minutes. Add two-thirds of the stock (which should be hot), and simmer until all the stock is absorbed. Add the mushrooms and the remaining stock and simmer until nearly all the stock is absorbed and the rice is tender and creamy. (If the rice is not tender, add more stock and simmer as necessary.)

Season to taste. Add the pine nuts, cheese and basil to serve.

TIP
- Don't use ordinary long-grain rice; it doesn't produce the correct risotto texture.

· *Ratatouille and Eggs in a Baked* · *Herb Crust*

Serves 4
220 calories; 12g fat per portion

1 tablespoon olive oil
2 medium onions, sliced
2 green peppers, de-seeded and
    sliced
1 medium aubergine, chopped
2 medium courgettes, cut into 1cm
    (1/2 in) rounds
2 cloves garlic, crushed
1 x 400g (14oz) can chopped
    tomatoes

1 teaspoon ground coriander seed
A little salt
Black pepper
4 size 3 eggs
50g (2oz) stale bread, chopped into
    tiny pieces
1 heaped teaspoon dried oregano
2 tablespoons Parmesan cheese

Heat the oil in a non-stick, lidded sauté pan or flameproof casserole and stir the onion over a medium heat for 5 minutes. Add the peppers and stir for 2 minutes. Add the rest of the vegetables, the garlic, tomatoes and coriander seed, stir, bring to simmer and cook, covered, for 1 hour. Season to taste.

Turn the ratatouille into four gratin dishes and make a dip in the centre of each. Break an egg into each dip. Mix the bread with the herbs and cheese and sprinkle over the dishes evenly. Bake at

200°C, 400°F, Gas Mark 6 for 20 minutes or until the eggs are just set and the topping is golden.

TIP

● If the breadcrumbs aren't stale they won't turn golden by the time the eggs are ready.

· *Gratin of Pulses and Vegetables* ·

Serves 4
270 calories; 7g fat per portion

1 tablespoon olive oil
1 large onion, sliced
2 sticks celery, chopped
1 clove garlic, crushed
2 medium carrots, cut into rounds
200g (7oz) squash (e.g., butternut or other orange-fleshed, firm pumpkin)
550ml (1 pint) vegetable stock
2 tablespoons tomato purée
100g (3^1/2 oz) dry weight brown lentils

50g (2oz) open-gill mushrooms
A little salt
Black pepper
75g (3oz) canned, drained chick peas
200g (7oz) can black-eye beans, drained *or* 125g (4oz) cooked beans
50g (2oz) bread, cut into very small pieces
50g (2oz) half-fat grated Mozzarella

Heat the oil in a sauté pan and stir-fry the onion, celery and garlic for a few minutes. Add the carrot and squash and stir for a few more minutes. Add the stock, tomato purée, lentils, mushrooms and seasoning and simmer, covered, for 30 minutes or until the lentils are tender, adding more stock if necessary. Add the chick peas and black-eye beans, and check seasoning. Turn the mixture into one large or four small gratin dishes and top with the bread mixed with the cheese. Grill under a medium heat for 7–8 minutes or until the bread is crisp and golden.

TIP

● If you can't get squash, a good alternative is sweet potato or swede.

· Buckwheat Pancakes with ·
Mushrooms and Cheese Sauce

Serves 4
395 calories; 14.5g fat per serving

1 quantity cheese sauce (see recipe, page 110)
50g (2oz) plain flour
50g (2oz) buckwheat flour
275ml (1/2 pint) skimmed milk
1 size 3 egg
A little salt

Black pepper
Fry Light spray
1 tablespoon corn oil
250g (9oz) chestnut mushrooms, sliced
1 tablespoon chopped parsley

Make the cheese sauce according to the recipe on page 110 and keep warm and covered. Beat together in a mixing bowl the flours, milk, egg and seasoning to make a light batter. Heat a heavy-based small frying pan (preferably one kept only for pancakes and omelettes) sprayed with Fry Light and, when very hot, use the batter to make eight pancakes. For each pancake, swirl a couple of spoonfuls of the mixture around the pan, brown the underside, turn and cook the other side for 30 seconds.

When each pancake is made, remove to a plate. When the eight pancakes are cooked, add the oil to another frying pan and when hot, add the mushrooms. Stir-fry them until reduced in size and turning golden; add the parsley and stir for a minute. Add half the cheese sauce to the mushrooms, stir well and then spoon one eighth of the mushroom mixture on to the centre of each pancake and roll up, tucking the ends in. Place the pancakes side by side in an oblong baking dish, pour the remaining cheese sauce over and bake at 200°C, 400°F, Gas Mark 6 for 20 minutes or until the sauce is bubbling.

TIP
● You can make the recipe using broccoli florets (lightly boiled) instead of the mushrooms.

· *Spiced Potato and Aubergine* ·

Serves 4
240 calories; 7g fat per portion

450g (1lb) old potatoes, peeled and cubed
1 large aubergine or 2 small ones
1¹/2 tablespoons corn oil
2 medium onions, sliced
1 clove garlic, crushed
1 teaspoon cumin
1 teaspoon curry powder
1 level tablespoon garam masala
1 x 400g (14oz) can chopped tomatoes

200ml (¹/3 pint) vegetable stock or as necessary
100g (3¹/2 oz) green beans, halved
1 tablespoon tomato purée
A little salt
Juice of half a lemon
140ml (5fl oz) natural low-fat Bio yogurt

Parboil the potatoes. Slice the aubergine into chunks, brush with half the oil and grill under a medium heat for 2–3 minutes each side. Heat the rest of the oil in a large non-stick lidded sauté pan and stir-fry the onion and garlic over a medium heat for 3–4 minutes. Add the spices and stir for 1 minute. Add the potatoes, aubergine, tomatoes, stock, beans, tomato purée and seasoning. Stir and simmer, covered, for 20–30 minutes or until the onion is soft and the sauce rich. Check seasoning. Stir in the lemon juice and yogurt, warm through and serve.

TIPS
● Serve with boiled rice or pitta bread
● Increase the quantity of spices if you like a hotter taste.

· *SALADS* ·

· *Baby Vegetable and Chicken Salad* ·

Serves 2
325 calories; 5g fat per portion

200g (7oz) cooked lean chicken, cubed
100g (3^1/2 oz) baby carrots, lightly boiled
75g (3oz) baby broad beans, lightly boiled
50g (2oz) petit pois, lightly boiled
6 cherry tomatoes
6 spring onions
200g (7oz) new potatoes, cooked and chopped if necessary

Dressing
3 tablespoons low-fat natural Bio yogurt
1 tablespoon Kraft 70% fat-free mayonnaise
1 dessertspoon lemon juice
1 dessertspoon fresh chopped parsley
A little salt and black pepper

Combine all the dressing ingredients in a small bowl. Combine all the salad ingredients in a serving bowl, pour the dressing over, lightly combine, and serve.

TIP
● You can use baby artichoke hearts, ready cooked, instead of the broad beans.

· *Pasta and Tuna Salad* ·

Serves 2
405 calories; 9g fat per portion

75g (3oz) dry weight pasta spirals
5 tablespoons oil-free French dressing
1 tablespoon olive oil
Pinch caster sugar
1 apple

200g (7oz) tuna in brine, drained
50g (2oz) cooked weight red kidney beans or butter beans
50g (2oz) sweetcorn, cooked
2 sticks celery, chopped
25g (1oz) raisins

Cook the pasta in plenty of lightly salted boiling water and drain. Combine the oil-free dressing with the olive oil and sugar. Chop the apple (but leave the skin on) and mix all the salad ingredients with the pasta and dressing.

TIP

● Red skinned apple looks nicest in this salad.

· *Ham, Egg and Potato Salad* ·

Serves 2
305 calories; 8g fat per portion

150g (5¹/2 oz) lean ham, chopped
1 size 3 egg, hard-boiled, shelled and sliced
250g (9oz) cooked waxy potato, cubed
2 tomatoes, de-seeded and chopped
2.5cm (1in) piece cucumber, chopped
Half bunch watercress, de-stalked
A few chicory or Chinese leaves, sliced
50g (2oz) beansprouts

Dressing
4 tablespoons 8% fat fromage frais
2 tablespoons low-fat natural Bio yogurt
1 tablespoon chopped chives
A little salt and black pepper

Combine all the salad ingredients in a serving bowl. Combine all the dressing ingredients in a small bowl and pour over the salad, mixing lightly.

TIP

● If your dressing is a bit too thick, add a little skimmed milk for a runnier consistency.

· *Cheese, Pineapple and Pasta Salad* ·

Serves 2
410 calories; 15g fat per portion

75g (3oz) dry weight pasta shells
50g (2oz) broccoli, cut into small florets
75g (3oz) Edam cheese, cubed
2 sticks celery, chopped
25g (1oz) sultanas
2 rings pineapple in natural juice, drained
1 small red pepper, chopped

1 tablespoon sesame seeds or pine nuts
4 tablespoons natural low-fat Bio yogurt
2 tablespoons 8% fat fromage frais
1 tablespoon chopped chives
A little salt and black pepper

Cook the pasta in plenty of lightly salted boiling water, adding the broccoli to the water for the last 3 minutes. Drain. Combine all the salad ingredients with the pasta and broccoli in a serving bowl. Combine the yogurt, fromage frais, chives and seasoning in a small bowl and pour over the salad. Mix well.

TIP

● Try chopped ready-to-eat dried apricots in the salad instead of sultanas.

· *Mixed Bean Salad with Fruit* ·

Serves 2
410 calories; 11g fat per portion

1 orange
1 tablespoon olive oil
3 tablespoons oil-free French dressing
Pinch caster sugar
200g (7oz) can mixed bean salad
50g (2oz) cooked green beans, halved

100g (3^1/$_2$ oz) cooked weight green lentils
50g (2oz) dry weight brown rice, boiled
1 banana
25g (1oz) chopped ready-to-eat dried apricot
mixed lettuce leaves

Peel the orange with a knife and cut it into segments reserving any juice from the orange as you do so. Combine the olive oil,

French dressing and sugar with the reserved orange juice in a small bowl. Combine all the other ingredients except the lettuce.

Arrange the lettuce in a serving dish. Mix the dressing and bean salad together and pile on to the lettuce.

TIP

● Chop the banana at the last minute to save it from going brown.

· *Provençal Salad with Goat's Cheese* ·

Serves 2
400 calories; 17g fat per serving

110g (4oz) medium-fat goat's cheese	mixed salad leaves
1 medium aubergine	1 tablespoon red wine vinegar
2 medium courgettes	1 dessertspoon balsamic vinegar
1 medium red pepper	Black pepper and salt
4 medium cloves garlic, in skins	1 teaspoon French mustard
1 tablespoon olive oil	A few sprigs fresh thyme
	150g (5^1/$_2$ oz) dark rye bread

Cut the goat's cheese into four. Slice the aubergine into rounds then quarters; slice the courgette into rounds, and de-seed and cut the red pepper into squares. Brush the aubergine with half the olive oil and arrange the vegetables with the garlic (the cloves left in their skins) on a baking tray. Bake for 30 minutes at 200°C, 400°F, Gas Mark 6.

Meanwhile, arrange the salad leaves on a serving platter, and combine the rest of the olive oil, the vinegars, seasoning, mustard and thyme in a small bowl. When the vegetables come out of the oven, squeeze the garlic flesh out of the skins and into the dressing. Mix well. Arrange the vegetables on the platter with the goat's cheese in the centre and drizzle over the dressing. Serve warm, with the rye bread.

TIP

● You can add a quartered beef tomato to the baking tray if you like.

· *Prawn Salad with Cashews* ·

Serves 2
460 calories; 18g fat per portion

50g (2oz) dry weight medium egg thread noodles
175g (6oz) good quality cooked shelled prawns
50g (2oz) mangetout, lightly cooked
1 slice canteloupe melon, cubed
1 banana
50g (2oz) mushrooms
25g (1oz) shelled, unsalted cashew nuts

4 spring onions
4 Chinese leaves, shredded

Dressing
1 tablespoon soya sauce
2 tablespoons lime juice
1 tablespoon sesame oil
1 tablespoon sesame seeds

Cook the noodles according to packet instructions and drain. Combine all the salad ingredients with the noodles in a serving bowl. Mix the dressing ingredients together and mix into the salad.

TIP
● Toss the banana into the dressing as soon as you have sliced it, to save it from going brown.

· *MISCELLANEOUS* ·

· *Fruit and Nut Compote* ·

Serves 2
255 calories; 2g fat per portion

75g (3oz) stoned ready-to-eat prunes
75g (3oz) ready-to-eat dried apricots
2 ready-to-eat dried figs, halved
200ml (7fl oz) orange juice
2 cloves
Pinch cinnamon

Pinch ginger
1 teaspoon grated lemon rind
A little water
1 fresh apple
175g (6oz) slice melon
1 tablespoon chopped nuts or seeds of choice

Put the prunes, apricots and figs in a saucepan with the orange juice, spices, lemon rind and a little water to cover. Simmer, covered, for 30 minutes or until all the fruit is tender, adding extra water if the mixture gets too dry, as you want plenty of nice juice. Chop the apple and melon and add to the compote with the nuts or seeds. Stir thoroughly and allow to cool before serving.

TIPS

- Use ready-to-eat dried fruits as they are tender and nicer than the old-fashioned type of dried fruit.
- The compote will keep for a few days in the fridge if in an airtight container. If you intend to eat it frequently you could double the quantities.

· *Spicy Rice Stuffing* ·

Serves 4
285 calories; 8g fat per portion

75g (3oz) dry weight bulgar wheat
75g (3oz) dry weight brown rice
$1/2$ teaspoon cardamom
$1/2$ teaspoon ground cloves
$1/2$ teaspoon cinnamon
Rind of half a lemon
75ml (3fl oz) orange juice

50g (2oz) chopped dried apricots
50g (2oz) sultanas
25g (1oz) sunflower seeds
25g (1oz) pistachio nuts, shelled, halved
Salt and pepper
2 tablespoons chopped parsley

Cook the rice until tender. Soak the bulgar as instructed on the packet. Mix the spices and lemon rind with the orange juice and combine with all the other ingredients well.

TIP

- Use the stuffing for filling vegetables to bake. Or used mixed with chicken, mushrooms, etc. for a supper dish, heated.

· *Cool Fruit Salad* ·

Serves 4
90 calories; trace fat per portion

200ml (7fl oz) apple juice
Juice of half a lemon
1 level dessertspoon fructose
1 green apple
200g (7oz) slice honeydew melon

1 small grapefruit
100g (3^1/$_2$ oz) seedless small green
  grapes
2 kiwifruit
Mint leaves

Combine the apple juice with the lemon juice and fructose. Wash the fruit if necessary and peel, chop, slice or segment as necessary. Add the fruit to the juice in a serving bowl, stir. Leave for an hour or two in the fridge and serve chilled, garnished with mint.

TIPS
- Vary the fruit if you like but try to stick to 'cool' colours such as green, white or pale yellow.
- The salad will keep a few days in a covered container in the fridge.

· *Cheese Sauce* ·

Serves 4
200 calories; 8.5g fat per portion

40g (1^1/$_2$ oz) low-fat spread
40g (1^1/$_2$ oz) plain flour
700ml (1^1/$_4$ pints) skimmed milk
1 level teaspoon dry mustard
  powder

Salt and black pepper
110g (4oz) half-fat hard cheese,
  grated

Heat the spread in a non-stick saucepan until melted and add the flour. Stir over the heat for a minute or two. Slowly add the milk (which should be warm) to the saucepan, stirring all the time. Add the mustard and seasoning when the sauce is thick and smooth, and lastly add the cheese, stirring until melted. Check seasoning.

6

WOMEN AND EXERCISE

'Tune into your body's own power and lose weight naturally.' That's the *Bodysense* promise which you read on the front cover.

And, when it comes to losing weight, *exercise* is your body's greatest natural source of power, and your body's greatest resource.

For, if you use your body as it was given to you to use, as it was made to be used, you will find slimming down to a natural weight much easier, and maintaining that weight very much easier, too.

Exercise is natural, and exercise is health-promoting. And, for women, especially, exercise brings so many extra benefits, it is almost unbelievable that a massive majority of us (between 60% and 90%, depending upon which reports you read) *still choose* to ignore this vital, natural source of power and well-being.

So *why* don't women take exercise?

I asked dozens of women that very question while researching this book. And here are some of the most typical replies:

'I know I am not fit but I'm frightened of finding out just how unfit I am. Ignorance is bliss.'

'Everyday life keeps me fit enough – I am always dashing around.'

'I would feel a fool starting an exercise class because everyone else will be slim and fit and I will not.'

'Part of me wants to exercise but I haven't a clue where to start. Also I've read that exercise is dangerous if you don't do it properly.'

'It's habit really, isn't it? You haven't done anything for years so it's hard to motivate yourself to start even though you know you should.'

'There just is no time even to think about exercising. All the women I know are just too busy with work and family. If I get any spare time I'd rather relax or see friends than go for a work-out.'

'Face it – exercise isn't enjoyable. It's a chore. We have enough chores in our lives without adding another.'

'Getting fit is vanity. When you talk about fitness it reminds me of Princess Diana going to her expensive gym every day in her designer wear. It's all right for her – but I'd feel guilty spending unnecessary time on myself.'

Phew! what an onslaught – but a real eye-opener too. I analysed all the answers I received and the objections to exercise seemed to fall into three main categories:

1 *Exercise is vanity;* a bit like dyeing your hair or painting your toenails. Many women feel that time spent on exercise is time when they should be doing something 'better' so they feel guilty. Yes, you say, maybe I'll get a flatter tum or burn off the calories in that cake I've just eaten – but there are so many more important things to do in life.

If that sounds like you, I can guarantee that by the end of this chapter you will have changed your mind.

Similarly, because the importance of exercise is lost to most of us, we say we 'have no time' to do it. Statistics show that more women than men give up regular exercise after they leave full-time education (before, if they possibly can!). Men continue to exercise at the weekends – playing team sports or golf, for instance, or cycling. And during the working week they often visit the gym or the pool before or after work.

Women will spend their time outside work shopping for food, child rearing, doing household chores – whatever. Men *do* have more spare time than women, on average. I don't see how anyone can argue with that. And so, because for most of us exercise is something of no great importance, and therefore we've got out of the habit of it, it is the easiest thing to forget about as we organise our busy lives. We say we've 'no time'. What we mean is, we don't want to make time.

We can always make time for something we really want to do. And, again, by the end of this chapter I think you *will* want to exercise. So you will find time.

2 *Exercise is disliked.* Blunt and stark, but true. Our negative feelings about exercise range from mild boredom, through serious

boredom, to memories of deep embarrassment last time we donned a pair of shorts or a leotard and on to deep fear – of hurt, of pain, of simply not being able to do it. And, of course, fear of discovering the real, poor state of our bodies.

A lot of negatives, there, then, to overcome. If you have some of those feelings, please do yourself a huge favour and blank your mind of them. Put a little trust in me and believe that exercise takes very many different forms and that one, or several, of those forms is going to be something that offers you *nothing* negative but *plenty* positive. Something suitable for you, and your body, and your confidence level, and your boredom threshold.

3 *Extra exercise is superfluous.* This was a surprise – that many of you feel you get enough exercise just going about your daily life. That walking your child to school or doing the vacuuming or shopping keeps your body in good shape and that therefore you have no need at all to do anything else. Nearly half of the women I talked to felt this was one of the main reasons why they don't do any formal exercise.

A friend of mine explained that she spent 20 minutes a day walking her child to and from school and that was plenty of exercise – '20 minutes three times a week is all you need!' she said. 'I know – I've read it.'

I persuaded that same friend to take a cardio-vascular fitness test and, as I suspected, her fitness rating was poor to moderate. She hadn't considered the fact that when she did the school walk with her five-year-old, she didn't do a 'proper' aerobic walk – more of an erratic dawdle, as her five-year-old walks very slowly, with the occasional anaerobic burst to dash after the child when she sees something of interest on the other side of the road. That's stress, not fitness training!

The truths are these:
- Exercise is perhaps the most wonderful provider of health insurance and well-being for women imaginable. It is not a waste of your time.
- To begin exercising takes motivation, but to exercise need not and should not be a negative experience if you go about it in the right way, and the right way *for you*.

- Exercise can be enjoyable.
- However active your daily life seems to be, the activity you get is probably not enough to give you optimum fitness.

Let's see how we can make exercise something you really want to do.

· *The Benefits of Exercising* ·
Your Body

First let's learn about all the marvellous things that happen when we exercise.

Exercise helps you to lose weight

All body movement burns up calories for energy, whether it is getting up from a chair, turning over in bed or walking downstairs.

But a normal, average diet of around 2,000 calories a day for women provides more than enough calories to replace all the energy used by our bodies in these ordinary, day-to-day movements. By building extra activity into your regular routine, you can burn off extra calories – enough to stop weight gain or, perhaps, even to create gradual weight loss.

Combine this calorie deficit brought about by increased activity, with a slight reduction in the amount of calories you consume, and you have an easy way to lose weight without having to cut back too much on the amount you eat.

As an example, an extra half hour a day of exercise that gets you slightly breathless – e.g., moderate walking – can help you to burn off an extra 900 calories a week or so, resulting in a weight loss of about 1lb (0.5kg) a month – or near enough a stone a year! Looked at that way, exercise has a great deal to contribute to your weight-loss programme.

Add to that a reduction in calorie intake of a mere 500 a day – from, say, 2,000 to 1,500, and (as 3,500 calories approximately equal 1lb (0.5kg) body fat) you have a weight loss of 5lb (2.5kg) a month (1lb (0.5kg) from exercise and 4lb (2kg) from eating less) – which adds up to more than four stones a year.

Exercise helps you to maintain your ideal weight for life

Once you've reached your target weight, if you continue to exercise regularly in the same way, you will be able to eat as much as – perhaps even more than – you did when you were overweight and not exercising, and maintain your new, trimmer shape. This works in two ways – aerobic exercise burns up calories for energy, and strength work builds up muscle which uses up more calories in your body than any other body component.

How much you can eat without getting fat if you increase your exercise levels depends, of course, on the amount of exercise you do – but for most of us, a little regular exercise is the key to weight maintenance even more than keeping a check on the calories.

Exercise may help you to live longer

All surveys on the subject show that people who keep themselves fit – or who get themselves fit at any age – live longer than people who don't exercise. One of the main reasons is that people who exercise have stronger, fitter, cardio-vascular (heart/lung) systems, less risk of high blood pressure and less risk of atherosclerosis (furring/hardening of the arteries) and stroke.

Exercise keeps everything in your body fit – and that includes things you may not have thought of.

Exercise will help you to a healthier old age

If you exercise, you'll enjoy a healthier old age in many ways. For example, exercise can help to control diabetes. Exercise helps to prevent osteoporosis (loss of bone density and susceptibility to fracture which is five times as common in women as it is in men). Exercise can help to minimise circulatory problems and keep you warm. Exercise can keep your joints mobile and reduce the problems associated with arthritis. It can even improve your hearing. And these are just a few of the benefits.

Exercise can give you a better-looking body

The right type of exercise can firm and tone you up, and can appear to slim you down where you need it, and even make you more shapely. Obviously, there are limitations, depending on your particular shape (see Chapter One), but exercise can do for you what your diet won't – fine tune the details! Exercise is so good at keeping you, literally, 'in good shape' that you may be able to maintain a higher weight than someone else of your body type and height, but look trimmer – and be able to wear smaller sizes in clothes.

Exercise also helps you to a better-looking body by improving your body alignment (posture) so that you stand better and, depending on what exercise you do, all kinds of bad body habits will gradually disappear. We'll be discussing body alignment later in the book.

Exercise helps to improve your sense of well-being

The right type of exercise increases the amount of oxygen that reaches all parts of your body, including your brain, and can make a positive difference to your mood, lifting sluggishness, vague tiredness or inertia. Exercise also releases endorphins which have a mood-enhancing effect.

Because of the increase in oxygen to the brain, exercise improves concentration, memory, mental agility and efficiency. In other words, an exercise session during a working day may literally work wonders for your capabilities in your job.

People who exercise generally have a healthier body image and more confidence than people who don't.

Exercise makes you stronger

The right type of exercise can help you to maintain sufficient muscular strength to help you considerably in your day-to-day life. Women are weaker than men physically for the simple reason that they don't have as much muscle. Most women don't want bulky muscles anyway, but it does help to make the most of what muscle we can develop, because a certain amount of strength really does help us to get through life more easily. Carrying shopping, lifting children, housework, gardening, stacking shelves, changing tyres or driving a lorry all require strength. There aren't many women around now who want to be 'girlies', standing around and hoping some strong man will arrive to sort everything out. And there are some tasks a man couldn't sort out for us even if we wanted him to, such as giving birth. If you're fit, pregnancy and the birth should be much pleasanter and easier – and of course your baby stands a better chance of being fit and healthy, too. (More on pregnancy in Chapter Eight.)

Being strong isn't just about having strong arm and leg muscles – if you strengthen your stomach muscles you will support your back and help to prevent backache throughout your life – something we could almost all do with, I reckon.

Exercise can help you to better sex

Exercise can improve your stamina – helping you to stay the course with your lover. And the right type of exercise helps to keep your pelvic floor muscles – and vagina – tight, and so will improve both your, and your partner's enjoyment.

Exercise will also help you to relax and feel good about your body, which, as every woman will admit, is a crucial part of enjoying intimacy with a partner.

Exercise helps you to relax

Not just for sex, but in many areas of your life, exercise as a reliever of stress and tension is a *very* important point. Men may moan about stress, but women tend to keep it bottled up and find it hard to wind down. You can be tired, exhausted even at the end of the day, but not relaxed. That's where your exercise session wins. When you've finished, you will always feel more relaxed, whether you've been walking or dancing, or have simply done a floor routine with plenty of stretching.

Hardly a surprise, then, that regular exercise can help you to a better night's sleep. And that, alone, for me makes exercise well worth doing.

Exercise helps your monthly cycle

Any woman who suffers from PMS, irregular periods or bouts of bingeing linked to her monthly cycle, wants all the help she can get – and exercise is a great way of helping by *natural* means.

Exercise helps in so many ways – it can help to bring on a period that is reluctant to start; it helps to keep fluid retention to a minimum, helps to control the urge to binge, helps to minimise stomach cramps and backache and helps to control mood and stress. So, exercise is essential for women in Phase Three of their cycie.

Yet many women do even *less* exercise than usual when they are suffering from PMS.

Exercise and women's health

Apart from helping to relieve PMS and in the prevention of osteoporosis, exercise also helps women to cope with, or prevent, other 'female' problems. The right exercise can minimise stress incontinence, especially after childbirth. It can also minimise the risk of prolapse (uterus or bladder sinking into the vaginal passage). And exercise can certainly help you through pregnancy and the menopause (see Chapter Eight).

So, here is your motivation: if your body is important and your life is important – then *so is exercise!*

· Finding the Time ·

But you still can't find the time to exercise? To begin with, you need to find only *two hours* a week (in small blocks to suit yourself).

Here's something to think about. You always manage to make time for certain things that happen in your life. Some expected, some unexpected.

- You make time for the extra work that Christmas involves each year.
- You make time to talk for an hour on the phone when your best friend rings and she is in a crisis.

- You make time to catch up on missed work when you have been ill.
- You make time to look after a parent, or a child, when he or she is sick.

Think of some more. If there is something you want to make time for, or you *have* to make time for – you do it.

Can you start thinking about exercise in the same way? To find the time may take a bit of lateral thinking, but it can be done. Here are some ideas:

- Get up a little earlier, especially if you are in the habit of waking and lying in bed.
- Re-organise your lunch break.
- Admit you could live without that TV soap you only watch out of habit. Or think of buying or begging an exercise bike and riding it while you watch.
- Persuade other members of your household to take a fairer share of the chores.
- Put some of those 'must do' chores lower down your priority list and put exercise up higher. For instance, exercise is definitely more important than perfect ironing or baking your own bread. It's more important than a spotless car, nail polish, reading a magazine, doing anything you don't want to do because you didn't like to say 'no' . . . and so on.
- Go to bed a little later to give you a little more time in the day. If exercise helps you to get to sleep more quickly and sleep more soundly, it won't matter.

Lastly, remember that exercise helps you to be more efficient, alert and happy, and thus it may save you more time than it takes! And remember that regular exercise is a habit that can become as second nature as, say, cleaning your teeth or having a cup of coffee – if you give it time.

· *Learning to Like Exercise* ·

So now let's move on to getting you started if you are a confirmed exercise hater. Let's take the most common reasons for hating exercise.

Embarrassment

The easiest way to prevent yourself from feeling embarrassed or foolish when you exercise is to begin exercising on your own. There is no law that says you have to visit a class or a gym or a pool. With the help of the next chapter you can begin to get fit and in shape on your own. And, maybe when you have lost your few pounds, or got into the hang of exercising, or feel a bit fitter, or more confident – then you can, if you want to, begin doing something more sociable. The important thing is to start, then see how you feel later.

But I must say a word here about that old 'embarrassment' question. Good leisure centres, good classes, good gyms, good teachers won't embarrass you anyway. Most classes are not full of superfit goddesses, anyway, but contain a fair proportion of people like you and me. And if you think you will be embarrassed because a routine or an instruction is too complicated, or an exercise too hard for you – then it is the class or gym, not you, who should be embarrassed.

If you ever do go to an exercise establishment where things don't seem right – complain, and/or stop going.

I must also point out that we are not all adept at the same things, physically. For example, you and a friend might decide to go to a beginners' aerobic class. She might pick up all the footwork first time while you may find the moves hard to follow. Or vice versa. The point then is to find something that does suit your own capabilities and preferences. Your friend may enjoy the aerobics class, but the fact is that you will become equally fit (maybe more so) by doing a Step class instead, or taking a brisk walk. There is no particular exercise you *have* to do to get you fit.

Boredom

Now let's move on to the familiar cry that exercise is boring. The truth is somewhat less of a sweeping statement than that. The truth is that all of us find some forms of exercise boring. But there is no need to do the type of exercise that bores you. Alternatively, make the exercise that you find boring, less boring.

For example, you may dislike floor toning exercises, but doing them to your favourite music may make all the difference. You may find walking boring – but if you walk with a friend that may make all the difference.

Probably it *is* those regular toning sessions that people find hardest to work up enthusiasm for and here I can only tell you what I do to get around this. I've never been a great fan of 'formal' 'set' exercise so I used two tricks to get myself to do them three or four times a week.

One, I knew from experience that if I did do them, I would *always* feel better afterwards – a sense of achievement and the glow that comes from having done something good for your body. So I set specific times aside to do the exercises and if I felt like saying 'no', I'd strongly visualise how I would feel afterwards, and this always did the trick. As I progressed, I began varying things by doing similar exercises in the swimming pool during my twice-weekly pool sessions.

Getting myself aerobically fit a few years ago (after years of doing virtually nothing) presented another problem. I lived 20 miles from the nearest decent aerobics class but had it been just around the corner I probably still wouldn't have gone as I am not, and never have been, someone who enjoys being part of a class or group. Instead, I chose footpath walking and, later, cycling. I love any exercise that involves some kind of visual pleasure.

The point is that at heart I am lazy and I am also quite busy – and if I could find ways of exercising, I know that you can too. I am not a natural 'exercise animal', and I don't think most of us are born athletes. But, as I said at the beginning of this chapter, our bodies *were* made to be used. And using them doesn't mean any one particular exercise form. Indeed, there is a lot to be said for variety, for doing several different things if boredom is your particular problem.

And once you start seeing results – a better body, fewer aches and pains, more stamina, and all the other benefits of exercise that I've described, doing it becomes easier and easier. You also get into the habit of fitting exercise in and it becomes second nature. Later on in this chapter, and in Chapter Seven, you will find much help towards making a programme to suit yourself. Use it!

Fear

You *can* do it. If you are in normal health, however unfit you are, you can get yourself much, much fitter; in shape and more supple and with better body alignment. The thing to do is take the little fitness test at the end of this chapter, then go slowly into your routine, gradually improving and *not comparing* yourself with anyone else.

Proper exercise involves *effort* but it shouldn't involve *pain* or even strong *discomfort*. It is absolutely untrue that exercise can only improve your fitness if you feel pain. So you need to learn the difference between a tired muscle and a muscle that has worked too hard. You need to know what level of 'puffed out-ness' when out walking is good and what degree is bad.

All this you will learn in the pages that follow so you should need have no fear about exercising at all.

Most of all, don't ever think, 'I'm never going to be able to do this.' The first session of any type of good exercise that you do, is *you* on the way to *your own* fitness. Yes, you may find certain moves in a floor routine hard (for instance, if you have very weak thigh muscles you will find the pliés on page 153 very difficult to start with) – but all that means is that you do need this exercise. And that if you keep trying, it will get easier and *you* will get stronger.

Keep looking at the results of exercise in *your* body. Keep remembering what it's all about.

I'm fit, I'm fine!

And lastly – so you think you already do enough exercise for fitness and health? That your busy daily life keeps you fit? Well, perhaps it does . . . but the chances of it doing so are quite small, unless you happen to be a professional sportsperson, or perhaps a PE teacher, or similar, in which case you probably won't be reading this book!

You can be 'on the go' all day, but still not improve your stamina – your heart/lung fitness. And take your mobility – how many times a day does your job require you to lift your arms above your head, or bend down to touch the floor? Try the three simple fitness tests at the end of this chapter and see how you do.

The fact is that modern gadgetry and convenience living has largely removed our need to use our bodies as much as they need to be used. So we must put that activity back into our lives by conscious means.

A reasonable level of fitness will actually help you to get through your day more easily and feel less shattered. So, don't tell me you're fit, you're fine as you are. Give it a go and see the difference.

· *How to Win at Exercise* ·

- Choose things you enjoy! If you try something once or twice and don't enjoy it, choose something else. (If you hate everything – you hate life!!)
- Don't choose anything too ambitious if you are unfit.
- If something bores you, don't give up exercising. Give up (at least temporarily) the thing that bores you and try something else. We all need variety. Or look at ways of alleviating the boredom. For instance, you could set yourself little goals. Chapter Seven contains exercise programmes with graduated goal suggestions; use these or similar ones of your own.
- Don't exercise to the point of hurting yourself. If you ache a lot the next day, you may not be doing the exercise right and/or not warming up or cooling down properly, or you may be doing something too hard for your current level.
- Go at your own pace.
- Don't like to sweat? Wear loose clothing and take a nice shower when you have finished. There is nothing wrong with perspiration – in aerobics, it is an indication (along with feeling warm) that you are burning calories.
- Don't think of exercise as punishment – it shouldn't feel that way. It's doing your body good and you should feel pleased to be doing it. If you are not (and you follow all the tips here), try to analyse why and alter the cause.

- Feeling tired and an exercise session is due? Remember exercise is an energy-giver and a mood enhancer, plus a relaxant. If you suit your exercise level to your mood and your phase, your session will help you to feel better, not worse.

    Be sensible – if you are truly exhausted, just a warm up and cool down with stretches may be enough for today.
- Don't do any vigorous exercise when you are ill.

· *Your Top Questions on Exercise* · *Answered*

There are so many different types of exercise – how do I know where to start and exactly what I need to do?

The fitness test that follows is the place to begin, followed by the *Bodysense* Ex-Plan in the next chapter. This offers what most of us need – some regular aerobic work (to strengthen your heart and increase your lung capacity, giving you more stamina), some tone and strength work (e.g., resistance exercises), and some flexibility work (for supple and mobile joints). At the end of this chapter, you will also find lists of 'symptoms', some of which your body may experience, listed with the correct type of exercise to cure that symptom. Use the test to help you to decide areas you need to do extra work on.

Is it a sensible idea to exercise with my partner? I think it might help to keep me motivated.

It could be, but you have to bear in mind that the average man (if your partner is male) will require a different type of exercise from the average woman in order to improve or retain fitness. Men are, on average, stronger than women and are likely to need a faster pace when building stamina, for example. Women, on the other hand, are often more flexible than men and better at exercise such as yoga, or at stretch sessions. Because of these differences it may not be easy to work out a routine that suits you both. However, you shouldn't have a problem in finding a female of similar fitness level to you, with whom you could exercise.

Is it okay to carry on exercising through my period?

Exercise helps to alleviate period symptoms such as stomach cramps and lower back pain. It also helps to lift your mood. So carry on exercising as far as is practical – there are more guidelines on Phase Three exercising in the next chapter.

What is the best way to build muscle? I've no definition at all in my legs and arms, though I'm not that thin.

Resistance exercises – using your own body weight, free weights, elastic resistance or gym equipment such as Nautilus – are best. You repeat each move just to the point where the muscle being worked is fatigued (tremor begins), then you stop. As you get stronger you increase the resistance. You will see quick results this way – but don't start using weights until you are familiar with body toning exercises done on their own. Aerobic activity such as walking or cycling will help to build shapely bottom and leg muscles.

I haven't exercised in years and I want to tone up, but I don't want bulky muscles. What is my best bet for exercise?

Most women are highly unlikely to build bulky muscle mass doing a normal amount of exercise because, as explained earlier, their bodies don't contain enough testosterone, the male hormone that facilitates muscle bulk building.

Female body builders work out, hard, several hours a day and have a genetic predisposition to build muscle. The amount of muscle you are likely to put on following resistance exercises or body conditioning – such as the basic plan in the next chapter – will be enough to produce a better shape and definition to your body but *not* the type of muscle that you feel looks unsightly. By the way – men and women who do no strength training lose approximately 5lb (2.5kg) of their muscle weight every 10 years after their 20s!

What exercise should I do in pregnancy?

Turn to Chapter Eight where you will find the answers.

Can you take up exercise at any age?

If you are in reasonable health, yes. But if you've never exercised and are over 40, I'd say talk to your doctor about what you would like to do. Regular walking and a few gentle toning exercises and stretches should be suitable at any age. Trials show that people who take up exercise later in life show as rapid improvement as young people.

Obviously, if you are 60 and have never exercised, you are not going to be able to get as fit as a 25-year-old in peak form. But that doesn't matter – very few of us will ever want to train to our maximum fitness, anyway.

How far should I go in the quest for fitness? How do I know when I am 'fit enough'?

It is easy to tell when you are *not* fit enough – try the three tests at the end of this chapter. But knowing when you are fit enough is largely a matter of common sense.

The *Bodysense* Ex-Plan, if followed as laid out, will give you adequate aerobic fitness, body tone and strength and flexibility for average, everyday needs. However, if you wanted to get fit enough to, say, be competitive at marathons, or climb mountains, then you would need to train further.

What you don't want to do is turn your interest in exercise into an obsession. 'Overtraining' can cause injury and burn out and can make your body more susceptible to viruses and illnesses. It can also stop your periods happening, which, long-term, is obviously not a good idea, especially if you want a family.

Remember: our bodies need rest.

· *The Bodysense Ex-plan* ·

The *Bodysense* Ex-Plan is not revolutionary; it contains no amazing new ideas or exercise routines; it will not work miracles. But it offers you what I think most women want from an exercise programme:

- It leads you to the areas and ideas that are right for you.
- It doesn't assume you know a lot, or have any current level of fitness.

- It allows you to build up gradually at your own pace.
- It offers leeway and guidance on exercising to fit in with the phase of your cycle, or your perceived phase.
- It offers a simple programme that you can fit around your life and your needs.
- If followed regularly, it will help to give you the many benefits of exercise described earlier in the chapter.

But before you begin, there are two important things left for you to do – first, take the fitness test that follows, and then use the symptoms check list to help you to pinpoint your own weakest areas.

· *Aerobic Fitness (Heart-Lung) Test* ·

The Step Test

For this test you will need a 20cm (8 inch) sturdy platform or step or stair plus a watch, comfortable clothes and training shoes. Warm up by walking on the spot for one minute.

Now stand in front of the step and step on and off it for three minutes. One complete step routine involves stepping up with your right foot, following with your left foot, returning your left foot to the floor; returning your right foot to the floor. You need to do approximately 20 complete steps per minute for the test to be accurate.

Do the stepping rhythmically, and at the end of three minutes (or earlier if you are gasping for breath, or your thigh, bottom or calf muscles are too weak to continue), look at the 'perceived effort' chart below, decide on your category, then read off the result underneath.

1 Very, very easy.
2 Very easy.
3 Easy.
4 Fairly easy.
5 Moderate.
6 Moderately difficult.

7 Hard.
8 Very hard.
9 Very, very hard.
10 Couldn't complete the test.

Result

1–3

You are very fit aerobically and will probably find the early stages of the *Bodysense* Ex-Plan aerobics too easy for you to gain any training effect from them. Start the programme at level 3 or 4.

4–6

You are moderately fit but could do with some aerobic improvement. You may find level 1 of the *Bodysense* aerobic plan too easy and can attempt level 2 straight away.

7–9

You are quite unfit and will reap great benefit from following the *Bodysense* aerobics plan in the next chapter. Begin at level 1 and take things at your own pace – but don't forget to try!

10

If you couldn't complete the test you are unfit – the shorter the amount of time you were able to carry out the stepping, the more unfit you are. Check with your doctor before beginning an aerobics plan and if given the go-ahead, work up to level 1 in your own time – for instance, by doing half the amount of walking suggested to begin with. If you are in reasonable health you will soon see rapid improvement in your fitness levels.

· *Body Strength* ·

Abdominal test

Lie on your back with hands at ears, and ankles crossed. Keeping legs still, raise head and neck off floor and curl in towards knees. Return to the floor. How many of these curl-ups can you do before tiring?

8 or less	Poor abdominal strength
9–15	Fair abdominal strength
16 or over	Good abdominal strength

Lower torso test

Lie on your stomache with your arms by your side. Breathe out and raise head and neck off the floor as far as they will go. How far off the floor does your chin go?

Less than 3 inches   Poor lower torso strength
3–6 inches   Fair lower torso strength
Over 6 inches   Good lower torso strength

Upper body test

Kneel on all fours with back straight, tummy tucked in, fingers pointing forward. Now slowly lower head towards floor, keeping it aligned with back. Slowly return to start. How many of these press-ups can you do before tiring?

8 or less   Poor upper body strength
9–15   Fair upper body strength
16 or over   Good upper body strength

Lower body test

Stand with feet hip-width apart and hands on upper front thighs. Lower your hips towards the floor until your thighs are at a 45° angle to the floor. Slowly raise to start. Do as many of these squats as you can in a controlled way. How many can you do?

8 or less   Poor lower body strength
9–15   Fair lower body strength
16 or over   Good lower body strength

The poorer your results in the strength tests, the more benefit you will reap from a tone and strength programme such as the *Bodysense* Ex-Plan, and from extra work if you can fit it in. Follow all the instructions in the next chapter.

· *Flexibility* ·

Shoulder test

Stand with feet an inch or two apart, knees relaxed. Clasp your fingers behind your back. Keeping your elbows bent, raise your arms out to the back as far as you can.

How far can you go (use a wall mirror to test your result)?

Hands hardly moved at all	Poor shoulder flexibility
Hands up to 6 inches away from back	Fair shoulder flexibility
Hands over 6 inches away from back	Good shoulder flexibility

Hamstrings and lower back test

Sit with right leg straight out, left leg bent and a little to the side. Keep your lower back straight, not curved, and move forward over the right leg as far as you can, reach your arms out and touch as far down your right leg as you can, without hunching your shoulders over. How far can you go?

No further than mid-calf	Poor hamstring and back flexibility
No further than ankle	Fair hamstring and lower back flexibility
To sole of foot or beyond	Good hamstring and lower back flexibility

If you did poorly in the flexibility tests, you will benefit greatly from doing the *Bodysense* Ex-Plan, and paying special attention to all the stretches both before and after the basic routine. Extra stretch work will help you to achieve better flexibility in a shorter space of time.

· *Symptoms Check List* ·

Your body symptoms and the exercise solutions

With the *Bodysense* Ex-Plan you will be working on each of the corners of the fitness 'triangle' – aerobic fitness, strength and tone, and flexibility. But we all differ in our ability in each area. For instance, you may be aerobically quite fit but have very poor flexibility. You may have good muscular strength but poor aerobic fitness. And so on.

This list helps you to identify your weaker areas, which as we've learnt throughout this chapter, have a far-reaching effect in many ways. Check down the symptoms on the left and tick which you feel apply to you. The right-hand column will then show you what type of exercise is most likely to cure or alleviate that problem or symptom. The more ticks you have in any one section, the more important it is that you fit in as much of that type of exercise as possible. Your options will be explained in detail in the next chapter.

Section 1

☐ Failed step test

☐ Pallor and poor skin tone

☐ Poor circulation – cold hands/feet

☐ Frequent sluggish feelings

☐ Slow weight loss despite sticking to eating plan

☐ Get out of breath easily

☐ Poor sleep patterns

☐ Fluid retention

☐ Constipation

☐ Pre-menstrual stress symptoms

☐ Mild depression

REGULAR AEROBIC ACTIVITY INDICATED

Section 2

☐ Failed strength test 1

☐ Failed strength test 2

☐ Failed strength test 3

☐ Flabby areas of body even if not overweight

☐ High waist to hip ratio (see Chapter One)

☐ Protruding stomach

☐ Low-slung bottom

☐ Muscular aches and pains

☐ Difficulty in lifting/carrying, e.g., small child/suitcase/shopping

☐ Poor posture result in section 6

☐ History of osteoporosis in family

☐ Endomorphic body type (see Chapter One)

☐ Ectomorphic body type (see Chapter One)

☐ Slow weight loss despite sticking to eating plan

BODY CONDITIONING AND STRENGTH EXERCISES INDICATED

Section 3

☐ Failed flexibility test 1
☐ Failed flexibility test 2
☐ Poor posture
☐ Muscular aches and pains
☐ Sedentary job
☐ Shoulder/neck tension

EXTRA STRETCHING EXERCISES INDICATED

Section 4

☐ Difficulty in taking a deep breath
☐ Tendency to hold breath
☐ Poor sleep
☐ Poor concentration
☐ Headaches
☐ Shoulder/neck tension
☐ Pain when shoulder/neck touched
☐ Pre-menstrual stress
☐ Nervousness/panic

RELAXATION EXERCISES INDICATED

Section 5

☐ Period pains
☐ Period slow to start

EXTRA PELVIC, STOMACH AND BACK RELEASE WORK INDICATED

Section 6

☐ Rounded shoulders
☐ Protruding stomach
☐ Ticks in section 3
☐ Excessive curve in lower back
☐ Knees turned inward or outward
☐ Flat feet
☐ Stance lopsided when viewed from front
☐ Frequent low back pain

BODY ALIGNMENT EXERCISES INDICATED

Now turn to Chapter Seven for the exercises and routines that will make up the right programme for you and your needs.

7

THE BODYSENSE
EXERCISE PLAN

The exercise plan in this chapter is one that any woman in good health can follow. The most important thing that I feel I have done is to offer a plan that is as *simple* as possible, because I know from my own experience that if you open a book and you see reams of complicated instructions, heart rates to be measured, distances to be worked out, and so on – it puts you off before you have even begun.

So with the help of *Kathryn Cullen, Fitness Professionals' Instructor of the Year 1995/1996*, I have stripped away every-thing except the essentials and what remains is, I hope, a plan that you will find easy to follow; that you can do in as little as two hours a week, and that, nevertheless, offers you enough flexibility so that you can improve at your own pace and never be bored. The plan consists of :

For everyone!

Aerobic: Three (increasing to four) sessions a week of walking; minimum 20 minutes each. (Alternatives to walking are offered as an option.)

Tone, strength and stretch: Three sessions a week, minimum 20 minutes each, of a simple floor routine. You can do this routine on alternate days to the walking, or on the same day.

Sample timetables for this basic routine appear on page 136. (Alternatives to this routine are offered as an option.)

Optional

Depending upon how fit you want to get, and what symptoms you ticked in the sections at the end of Chapter Six, you can add on these optional extras:

Extra aerobics: Once you have completed the level 6 walking plan (or options to walking) as laid out in this chapter, you will be fit enough to add on extra aerobic work. Indeed, if you simply continue to repeat level 6 indefinitely, your aerobic fitness will remain static. Extra aerobic work you can do is detailed on page 140. If you ticked many of the boxes in Section 1 (page 131) you may gain even more benefit than other people from getting in plenty of aerobic work (though you should work through the six levels at your own pace before taking on extra).

Extra tone and strength exercise: Once you have mastered the basic tone and strength floor routine in this chapter you can do extra work as described on pages 172–3. This will ensure that you continue to improve. If you ticked many of the boxes in Section 2 (page 131) your body will definitely benefit from this extra work.

Extra stretch and relax: If you ticked many of the boxes in Sections 3 or 4, you will benefit from adding on the four extra stretches that appear on pages 173–4, to your basic routine. This will only take an extra two minutes.

Extra pelvic, stomach and lower back release work: If you ticked Section 5 on page 132, you will benefit from adding on the four extra exercises which appear on pages 174–6, during your Phase Three (just before your period and during the first two days of your period). These will only take 2–3 minutes to do.

Extra body alignment exercises: If you ticked many of the boxes in Section 6 on page 132, you suffer from poor body alignment and posture and will benefit from doing the extra body alignment exercises that appear on pages 176–8. These will take you 2–3 minutes.

When to do your extras:
If you do decide to do any of the extra work, it is best simply to add it on to the end of your basic 20-minute tone, strength and stretch routine as you will already be warmed up.

The only exception to that is extra aerobics work, which should, of course, be added on to your aerobic workout.

Exercise and the three phases

It is always a good idea to begin any new exercise plan (whether aerobic or toning) during a time when you feel good, positive and well. This means you will probably want to start during Phase One. If, like many women, your three phases coincide with the rhythm of your menstrual cycle, then this is the type of pattern that may be apparent:

PHASE ONE: Go for it! You feel strong, motivated. Towards the end of Phase One, at ovulation, research shows that women are at their absolute strongest and most creative (probably because of the high levels of oestrogen in your body at this time) so make the most of this to really progress with your programme. Phase One is a good time to move up a level in your aerobics routine – two, even – or to add on an extra set of repeats for your toning routine.

PHASE TWO: Directly after ovulation, Phase Two begins and this is the time to consolidate all the progress you have made during Phase One. You may well be able to make further improvement, especially in 'fine tuning' – for example, in performing a move in the floor routine perfectly for the first time; or in carrying through a stretch that little bit further.

PHASE THREE: The days leading up to your period and when your period begins. Time to be kind to your body by giving it the exercise it needs and not neglecting your body work. But don't expect quite so much of your body at this time. This is a good phase in which to do extra relaxation work and don't forget the pelvic exercises if you ticked Section 5. Stay on whatever level you achieved during your last phase until you return to Phase One after your period begins.

In Phase Three, it really is important to keep exercising. All research shows that exercise is beneficial pre-menstruation. Obviously, if you have a heavy period it may not be practical to do a long walk, but you can do one or two shorter walks. Remember that on days when you don't feel great, exercise may be the best cure. However, don't exercise if you are ill. Your body will need time to rest in order to fight the illness and recover.

Some schedule suggestions

I want the programme to be flexible so that it fits in with your life, so it is up to you to decide when to do your three 20-minute aerobic sessions and your three 20-minute toning sessions. But to help you you will find two sample programmes below. The only rule is not to do your toning three days in a row, then nothing for four days. These sessions need to be spaced out with rest days in between so that your muscles can recover properly. There are some tips and footnotes later in the chapter to help you to plan to optimum effect.

Suggested Schedule One
For women who prefer to do a little work every day:

A = Aerobics   T = Toning

	day 1	2	3	4	5	6	7
level 1	A–20	T–20	A–20	T–20	A–20	T–20	Rest
2	A–20	T–20	A–30	T–20	A–20	T–20	Rest
3	A–30	T–20	A–30	T–20	A–30	T–20	Rest
4	A–20	T–20	A–30	T–20	A–30	T–20	A–20
5	A–30	T–20	A–30	T–20	A–30	T–20	A–20
6	A–30	T–20	A–30	T–20	A–30	T–20	A–30

Suggested Schedule Two
For women who prefer to work on only three or four days of the week.

	day 1	2	3	4	5	6	7
level 1	A–20 T–20	Rest	A–20 T–20	Rest	A–20 T–20	Rest	Rest
2	A–20 T–20	Rest	A–30 T–20	Rest	A–20 T–20	Rest	Rest
3	A–30 T–20	Rest	A–30 T–20	Rest	A–30 T–20	Rest	Rest
4	A–20 T–20	Rest	A–30 T–20	Rest	A–30 T–20	Rest	A–20
5	A–30 T–20	Rest	A–30 T–20	Rest	A–30 T–20	Rest	A–20
6	A–30 T–20	Rest	A–30 T–20	Rest	A–30 T–20	Rest	A–30

· *Your Aerobic Routine* ·

There are six levels of aerobic activity through which you should gradually work your way. And, if you start on the easiest level and work your way up, there is no chance of doing too much and risking injury. Up to Level 3 you will be working aerobically three times a week, from Levels 4 to 6, four times a week. You may find that you can move through the levels at the rate of one a week so that you are on Level 6 by Week Six. However, there is no obligation to do this and you may stay on each level for two or more weeks if you like, or need to. However, there is no great advantage in staying on the same level for longer than you need. During Phase Three it is wise to stay on the same level – or even, if necessary, regress a level.

Walk to fitness

The aerobics routine I have chosen as optimum is a walking routine. This is for several reasons. To increase your heart strength and lung capacity (your cardio-vascular or aerobic fitness) and therefore your stamina, you need to do regular sessions of aerobic activity. Several activities are classed as aerobic but by far the most simple, probably the safest, most convenient and cheapest is walking.

And, for women who haven't exercised for a while, it is also the least daunting because you can do it on your own (or with a friend of similar fitness to yourself if you prefer); you can do it whenever and wherever you like, using clothes and shoes you probably already possess, and, of course, we all walk in our everyday lives (albeit not often aerobically), so we've got the basic knowledge of the art there already!

If you would rather do a different aerobic exercise than walking, then you can substitute your own chosen aerobic activity into the schedule. For suitable alternatives, turn to the 'Alternatives to Walking' section on page 141.

The right way to walk

To increase your cardio-vascular fitness, your walking needs to raise your pulse rate to a 'training' level and, because of this, many aerobic routines are accompanied by complicated heart-rate tables, training zone tables, and the like, which require you to take your pulse accurately and frequently. These charts are, for many of us, yet another reason never to begin and, for that reason, I'm not including them.

The fact is that, if you have a modicum of common sense you can work out whether or not your pulse rate is raised sufficiently to be giving you a training effect.

Quite simply, you are training at a suitable level when your breathing is noticeable and deeper, so that you feel moderately 'puffed' and you feel as though you are working. You should not be so puffed out that you can't talk, nor working so hard that you feel pain or undue stress, or have to stop. But an aerobic walk is *not* a 20-minute dawdle round the shops, either. Kathryn has worked out for you her own unique version of the 'perceived effort' test to help you decide whether you are working aerobically, or not. Look at the list below. You already know what the effort involved in each of her examples feels like. Well, a suitable training level for your walk should feel like number 5, 6 or 7.

Kathryn's Perceived Effort Chart

1   Lying in bed.
2   Window shopping.
3   Hanging the washing out.
4   Mowing the grass (powered mower).
5   Walking up one flight of stairs.
6   Walking to work if you're late.
7   Trying to catch up with someone walking faster than you.
8   Climbing up a long flight of steep stairs.
9   Sprinting for a bus.
10 Total exhaustion.

If your walk is no better than three or four, it isn't doing your aerobic fitness any good. Speed up a bit. If it is as hard as 8, 9 or 10, it is too hard; slow down a bit.

This training level should be kept up for a minimum of 15 minutes (at Level 1) up to 25 minutes (at Level 6). For the rest of your aerobic walking time, you should be warming up and cooling down. But Kathryn points out that if you are unfit, you can work up to a constant 15 minutes' aerobic walking (at Level 1) by doing a few minutes at perceived effort 6 or 7, then slowing down to around 4 or 5, then speeding up again to 6 or 7, until you can work at 6 or 7 all the time.

Warming up

Warming up consists of a few marches on the spot with arm movement at home before you leave, then use the first 2–3 minutes of your walk to slowly increase the pace, until you reach 4 or 5 on the Perceived Effort Chart, followed by short stretches to prepare your leg muscles for the workout. (See The Warm-up on page 147.) These should be 8-second stretches of numbers 1 to 7 on pages 148–151.

If you don't warm up you could risk injury to cold muscles, and stress to yourself.

Cooling down

Cooling down consists of spending the last 2–3 minutes of your walk gradually easing off the training pace so that you walk slower and your heart rate and breathing return to normal. By the time you arrive home you should be strolling. If your walk has made you sweat and/or you've peeled off layers as you walked, put something warm on again and do the long leg stretches 1–10 on pages 167–172 This will only take a few minutes and will help to ensure that you feel no aches or pains tomorrow – and this is the best time to increase mobility around your joints, too.

Now take a warm bath or shower; you deserve it!

Footnotes

● Many walking plans will give you a set distance to be covered in your allotted time. I have decided, with Kathryn's approval, that this isn't strictly necessary because, if you follow the commonsense guidelines above for exercising within your training zone, you will automatically be walking more quickly – and therefore covering more distance – as the weeks and levels progress. Also, at the higher levels, the time you spend

on your walk increases from 20 to 30 minutes, thus offering
more walking time.

The reason you will automatically walk further in the same
time if you are training correctly, is that as your heart and
lungs get slowly fitter, you will need to do more work to reach
that stage of moderate 'puff' that we talked about. More work,
in walking terms, means either walking more quickly or
perhaps walking uphill, which is another alternative.

- If you have chosen to do your toning routine on the same day
  as your walk, and you are going to do it at the same time of day
  rather than opposite ends, do your toning routine after your
  walk. This will save you time as you needn't then do the pre-
  toning warm up, but just go straight into the pre-toning
  stretches on page 148. Also, as you will be very nicely warmed
  up from the walk you will probably perform the exercises
  better and more easily.

- Style of walking is important. You need to pay attention to
  your posture – keep your stomach held in and walk from your
  hips. Keep your neck long; not hunched into your shoulders.
  Lift your ribcage up, keep shoulders relaxed down and pressed
  together. And keep your ears over your shoulders! As you
  speed up, you may use more natural arm movement to
  counterbalance your body.

- The six-level programme assumes you start off not very fit (but
  if you did well in the step test on page 127 you may start on a
  higher level than 1). Once you are doing Level 6 easily you
  should be fit enough for everyday life but you may want to
  improve further . . .

Extra aerobic work

Level 6 offers more training effect than may at first be apparent.
That is because you can continue to walk at a faster and faster
pace to produce the training effect, until, one day, you just can't
walk any faster without breaking into a run. If your joints are
supple, arthritis isn't a problem and you have a good pair of
supporting, cushioned shoes, you can, of course do exactly that –
start interval training – walking, then jogging a minute or two,

increasing the time spent on jogging with every week. So that is one way to get extra training effect.

Another way is to work for longer at each session. Instead of 30 minutes, do 45 minutes.

A third way is to do more uphill work or use harder terrain – sand or rough grass are harder to walk on than a smooth surface.

A final way is to do extra sessions of other aerobic activities – say, fit in a 20- or 30-minute session on day 6 of cycling, swimming or dance aerobics class. For more information and ideas on this, read the next section, 'Alternatives to walking', combined with the chart on pages 142–3.

- Kit: You don't need any special gear except comfy sweatpants and shirt, a light waterproof top, socks and comfortable, supportive walking shoes. These can be either aerobic trainers (preferably good quality ones) or cushioned walking boots such as Caterpillars. You might like to take along a flask of water or diluted orange juice with you, too, especially if the weather is hot.
- Don't walk alone in isolated areas especially in the dark. A companion of similar fitness level is a good idea. (A companion of a different fitness level will cause problems for your training.)

Alternatives to walking

If you don't want to walk, you can choose another aerobic activity instead, though if you are unfit I do advise walking as the best starting point at least for a few weeks.

The activity chart that appears on pages 142–3 rates many common activities (not just sports but all kinds of things like housework and gardening) from one star to three stars for aerobic training effect.

One star means the activity has little or no aerobic training effect (e.g., yoga). Two stars means there is moderate capacity to achieve aerobic training and three stars means this is an excellent activity for aerobic training.

The last column on the chart refers to the degree of difficulty of the activity, so that you can pick an activity that suits your current fitness level. If you are unfit and want an equivalent activity to do instead of walking on the early levels of the programme, you would choose a one-star activity such as slow dancing or grass mowing. Later you could choose a three-star rating for difficulty, such as hi-lo aerobics class, roller blading or rowing.

What you have to remember is that for a real training effect, you need to maintain the activity at a constant level for at least 15 minutes, up to 25 minutes at Level 6. If you are unused to the activity concerned, you may find this much harder than training walking. Skipping, for instance, is a wonderful training activity but extremely hard to do for more than even a minute if you are a beginner.

Perhaps, then, you could design a 'circuit' of your own lasting 20–30 minutes in all (depending upon which level you are on). This could be, say, three minutes marching on the spot, three minutes stair climbing, one minute skipping, all repeated three times. As long as you maintain your training level for 15 minutes (during 20 minute-sessions) or 25 minutes (during 30-minute sessions) that is fine.

Remember, if something is too hard and you can't maintain that training level, it won't work. Do something easier and come back to it when you are fitter; or do it in very small 'doses' as part of a complete routine.

· *Activity Chart* ·

Activity	Aerobic	Strength/tone		Flexibility	Cals per min used	Rating
		upper body	lower body			
Hi/lo aerobics	***	**	***	**	8	**
Beginners Aerobics class	***	**	***	**	7	*
Archery	*	**	*	*	3	*
Badminton	**	**	**	**	5	*
Basketball	**	**	**	**	5	**
Body conditioning class	**	***	***	***	4	*
Bodysense Strength and Stretch Programme	*	***	***	***	3	*

Activity	Aerobic	Strength/tone		Flexibility	Cals per min used	Rating
		upper body	lower body			
Circuit training (in gym)	***	***	***	**	5	**
Cricket	*	**	**	**	3	**
Cycling	***	*	***	*	7	**
Dancing (slow)	**	*	**	**	4	*
Dancing (disco or Latin type)	***	**	**	**	5	*
Digging	*	**	**	*	4	**
Fencing	**	**	**	*	5	**
Football	**	*	**	**	5	**
Golf	**	**	**	**	4	*
Gymnastics	**	***	***	***	5	**
Handball	**	**	***	**	4	*
Hockey	**	**	**	**	5	**
Horse riding	*	**	***	**	4	*
Housework	*	**	**	**	4	*
Ice skating	**	*	***	**	4	**
Jogging	***	*	***	*	7	***
Judo	*	**	**	***	4	**
Mowing grass (push-along mower)	**	**	**	*	5	*
Rock climbing	**	*	***	**	4	**
Roller skating	***	*	***	**	5	**
Rowing	***	***	**	*	7	***
Rugby	**	**	**	**	6	**
Running	***	*	***	*	8	***
Skiing, cross country	***	***	***	**	8	***
Skiing, downhill	**	**	***	**	6	**
Skipping (rope)	***	**	***	**	6	***
Squash	**	**	***	**	10	***
Stair climbing or stepping	***	*	***	*	8	**
Stretch classes	*	*	*	***	3	**
Swimming	***	***	***	**	7	**
Table tennis	**	**	**	**	5	*
Tennis	**	**	***	**	6	**
Volleyball	**	**	**	**	5	*
Walking	***	*	***	*	5	*
Weight lifting	*	***	**	*	7	***
Yoga	*	*	*	***	3	**
Yomping (alternating walk with jog)	***	*	***	*	6	**

And, lastly, remember that if your chosen activity one day no longer gets you 'puffed' enough to be having a training effect, it's time to do something harder – or else give yourself a pat on the back and say, 'Right, that's it now – I'm fit enough; I'm simply going to maintain my current level of fitness.'

And for how to do *that*, you need to read Chapter Eight, Bodysense Through Life.

· *Your 20-minute Tone, Strength* · *and Stretch Routine*

This programme will increase your body tone, strength and flexibility in as little as one hour a week. The three, 20-minute sessions will consist of:

● FIVE MINUTES warm-up and short stretches
● TWELVE MINUTES toning and strength exercises
● THREE MINUTES cool-down stretches.

The routine is as simple as Kathryn can make it while still working all the major muscles in your body. Timings for the routine are approximate, and obviously if you are just starting out, it may take you a little longer as you learn the moves, and as you get stronger over the weeks and begin to do extra sets of the toning and strength exercises, you will need a few more minutes. But it is important that you don't try to save time by skipping the warm-up or you will find the exercises harder to do and you will risk injuring yourself. And it is equally important not to rush the tone and strength exercises which need to be done in a controlled way to be effective, or the stretches which, apart from helping your body to become more flexible, also act as your cool-down and, may help to relieve potential aches and pains as well as improving your posture and balance.

Alternatives to the 20-minute routine

If you really don't want to do the Bodysense Tone, Strength and Stretch routine at all (though I think you will enjoy it if you do), use the Activity Chart on page 142–3 to find suitable substitutes. You will notice that all activities are rated from one to three stars for upper and lower body strength and flexibility. Choose any activity – or combination of activities that offer(s) good benefits. For example, swimming is good for upper and lower body strength *and* flexibility, so it is ideal. It is also a good aerobic exercise, so it's perfect for anyone who is short of time as you wouldn't need to do a separate aerobic programme on swimming days.

Tips

Before you begin, read these tips.

- Do the exercises at an optimum time of day for you – i.e., not when you are extremely tired or only half-awake.
- Don't do them when you are ill.
- Don't do them within one hour of a main meal, otherwise you may feel a bit nauseous.
- Breathe naturally throughout the exercises (breathing out as you exert yourself to do each move makes the exercise more effective).
- Wear light-to-warm, comfortable clothing that isn't restrictive but isn't too baggy, either, as you want to be able to see what your body is doing. Wear light, flexible trainers and socks.
- Wear a sweatshirt to warm up in, and after cool-down.
- Music may help you to enjoy the routine and perform it more rhythmically, but only if the beat of the music you choose matches your ability. If it is too fast, you will hurry your movements and do them poorly – faster doesn't mean better. If performed correctly, the slower and more controlled your movement, the harder it is.
- Do the exercise on a firm but softish, non-slip surface, e.g., a carpet with a towel or exercise mat on it, in a warm room. If you are cold, take longer over your warm-up until you feel truly warm.
- Unplug the phone and avoid interruptions; this is *your* time.
- Concentrate on what you are doing; don't daydream. Go through the routine twice, slowly, before you begin your first 'real' session. If possible, check in a mirror that your posture

looks like Kathryn's in the photos. Or ask a partner or friend to check it out for you. If you are not used to exercise, you will find it hard to perform each exercise exactly as shown in the photos at first. For instance, if you have weak abdominal muscles or an inflexible back, you will find it hard to come up off the floor as much as Kathryn is doing in the Curl Up. And if you have stiff, inflexible hamstring muscles, you will find the hamstring stretch very difficult at first.

But the whole point of this programme is to improve your body so if you try your best and concentrate, and do extra work on your weaker areas (in strength) and tighter areas (in stretch) you will gradually improve until you, too, can do everything perfectly, or nearly so.

It is better to do an exercise 'half way' than to find a way of doing it that is incorrect. That is why you must pay attention to the written instructions, and study the photos carefully to see what you're aiming for.

- Unless otherwise stated, the correct standing position for carrying out any of the standing exercises is: stand with legs shoulder-width apart, knees relaxed. Pull tummy in, tilt pelvis so that tailbone points directly to the floor. Keep buttocks relaxed and ribcage lifted, with shoulders pressed back and down. Lengthen neck and keep ears in line with shoulders. Check your position in a mirror.

Improving

It will probably take you several weeks simply to master the routine and do each exercise correctly and well, doing all the repeats mentioned and holding all the stretches for the right length of time.

When you have achieved that, it is time to think about improving.

This you can do by increasing the number of sets you do of each toning and strength exercise. You will, over the weeks, have built up to the recommended 12 repeats of each exercise, which is one set.

When you can do one set well with no muscle fatigue setting in at the end of the 12 repeats, try two sets (with a 15-second pause between sets). This will take you longer – but, as your proficiency has improved you will be carrying out the moves a little faster, so it won't take you that much longer to do extra sets.

You don't have to add on a complete, 12-repeat set of each move straight away – you can build up to a whole set, doing, say, four extra repeats to start with and working up to the full set of 12.

You can improve at stretching by doing the stretch better (i.e., with better body alignment), by stretching for longer, and by relaxing into your stretch.

Warm-up and short stretches (5 minutes)

1   To warm up, stand with legs slightly apart, knees relaxed, pull tummy in, and shrug your shoulders up and down 10 times; then forward and back 10 times. Now do circles to the front and then to the back.

2   March on the spot for 30 seconds, arms moving naturally, lifting feet an inch or two off the floor.

3   March for another 30 seconds, but this time with your knees lifted higher but not so high that your thighs go beyond parallel to the floor, or that your posture suffers.

4   Bring your legs further apart and continue marching for one minute, keeping your legs this far apart, bringing in plenty of natural arm movement.

5   Bring your right leg, with knee bent, across your body and up, bringing left arm down slightly to meet knee. Return right leg to floor and repeat the knee lift with your left knee. Continue for 30 seconds.

6   With feet a few inches apart, bring right lower leg up behind you into a hamstring curl so that your heel comes up behind you as high as it will go. Return to floor and repeat with left lower leg. Repeat for one minute, as rhythmically as you can, lifting your arms up and out from your sides as you go. Now you should feel warm, so it's on to the stretches.

Each of these stretches is a single movement which should be held for eight seconds. They should all be carried out standing up. Exercises 1–7 on pages 148–51 can be used as warm-up stretches for your aerobics programme.

WARM-UP STRETCHES

1 Back stretch
Stand with your
knees bent, palms on
thighs.

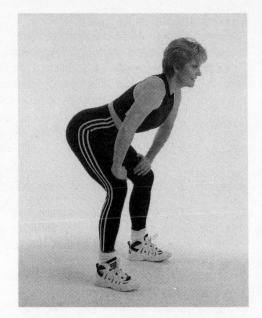

Curve the spine and
stretch out your back
as shown, feeling
your abdomen
pulling up in towards
your spine.

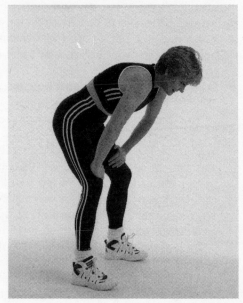

2 Side stretch
Stand with feet shoulder-width apart and keep knees soft. Place right hand halfway down right outer thigh for support and, taking care not to twist body to left or right, stretch up and over to the right, with left arm outstretched as shown. Feel the stretch along your left side. Return to the start and repeat on the other side.

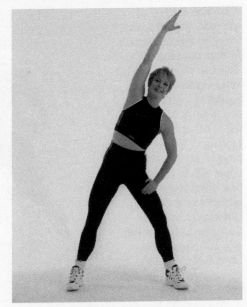

3 Hamstring stretch
Stand with legs together. Now slide your right foot forward and bend your left knee, leaning your body forward and resting your hands on your left thigh as shown. Lean forward from the hips and lift your tailbone up until you feel the stretch up the back of your right thigh. Repeat the stretch for your left leg.

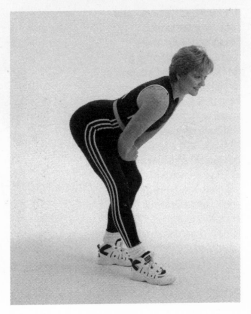

4 Combined upper calf and front shoulder stretch
Step your right leg approx. 45cm (18ins) behind your left leg as shown. Bend left knee over shoelaces. Straighten right leg with heel to the floor and both feet pointing forwards. Leaning body slightly forward, feel a stretch in upper calf. At the same time, clasp your hands behind your back with elbows bent, and raise your arms as high as they will go, keeping chest lifted. Feel the stretch across front of shoulders and a little in your chest.

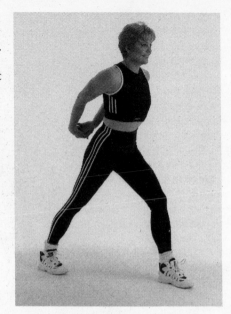

5 Combined lower calf and back shoulder stretch
Stand with your knees slightly bent, right leg a few inches behind left leg as shown. Bend right knee, keep heel to the floor. Feel a stretch in lower right calf and back of ankle (achilles tendon). At the same time, bring right arm across chest as shown and, using your left hand, gently press right elbow to stretch out right shoulder. Repeat complete stretch on other side.

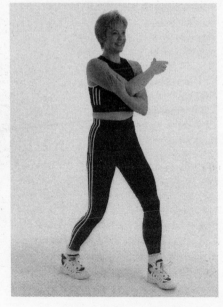

6 Quadriceps stretch
Stand with knees relaxed; lift right leg as shown, keeping right knee still and bringing right heel in towards your bottom with the help of your right hand (but don't force it). Press the top of the pelvis back. Feel the stretch up the front of your right thigh. Repeat for the left thigh.
TIP: For more support, rest your hand on the back of a chair.

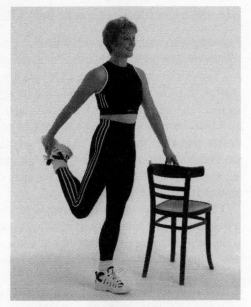

7 Inner thigh stretch
Stand with your feet wider than shoulder width apart, toes forward, knees slightly bent. Take your body weight over to your right leg and extend your left leg as shown, keeping your torso upright, until you feel a stretch along your inner left thigh. Repeat the stretch for the right leg.

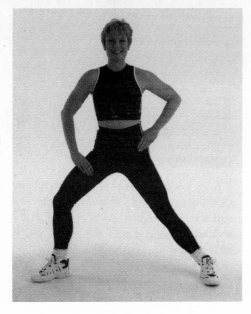

Strength and toning exercises (12 minutes)

Your aim is to complete one set of each of these exercises. One set comprises 12 repeats of the complete exercise movement. At first you may not be able to manage 12 repeats – indeed, you may only manage three or four. You should do as many repeats (up to 12) as you can, until the point of muscle fatigue – that is, the point at which the muscle being worked begins to tremor. Do not try to continue after that point. Stop that exercise and move on to the next exercise (or repeat on the other side if you are doing an exercise which involves working both sides of the body separately).

You should not stop an exercise until you have done all 12 repeats *unless* you have reached muscle fatigue.

In the weeks ahead you can add on extra sets of each exercise (see 'Improving' on page 146), in which case you should rest at least 15 seconds between sets.

You may not be able to do each exercise well at first, but try your best and concentrate, keep thinking 'slow' and 'control' and you will soon be excellent.

REMEMBER

Unless otherwise stated, the correct standing position for carrying out any of the standing exercises is: stand with legs shoulder-width apart, knees relaxed. Pull tummy in, tilt pelvis so that tailbone points directly to the floor. Keep buttocks relaxed and ribcage lifted, with shoulders pressed back and down. Lengthen neck and keep ears in line with shoulders. Check your position in a mirror.

STRENGTHEN AND TONE EXERCISES

1 Plié squats (for front and inner thighs, hip and bottom)
Stand with feet wider than shoulder width apart in correct pelvic position.

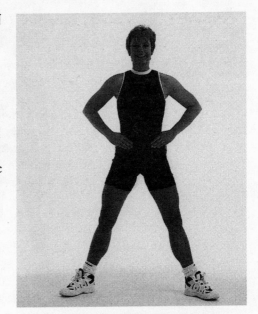

Bending your knees, lower your bottom into a squat (or as far as you can go). Slowly raise to start and repeat 12 times. **TIP:** keep your body as upright as possible and knees directly over shoelaces when you squat.

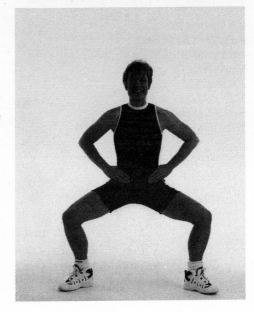

2 Parallel squats (for thighs, hips and bottom)
Stand in correct starting position (see page 146).

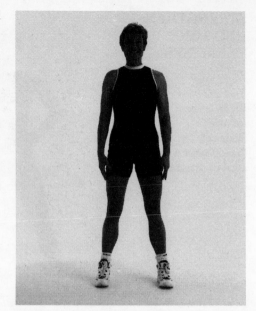

Slowly bend knees and hips to a 90° angle (or as far as you can go) and sit back. Slowly return to start and repeat 12 times. **TIP:** Your back will be at a diagonal angle to the floor.

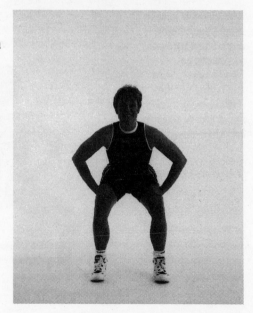

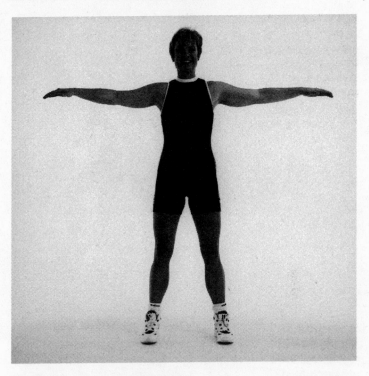

3 Lateral arm raises (for shoulders)

Stand in correct starting position (see Parallel squat on page 154). With arms at sides, face palms into body, thumbs pointing forward. Slowly raise both arms out and up to shoulder height, then slowly lower back to start. Repeat 12 times.

TIPS: Don't hunch your shoulders up as you do this. In later weeks you can add weights to increase the difficulty, starting with maximum 1kg (2lb) each hand.

4 Bent over row (for back)
Stand with your left leg forward of your right, left hand resting on mid left thigh. Lean forward over the left leg. Now bring your right arm forward, straight, in front of your right leg.

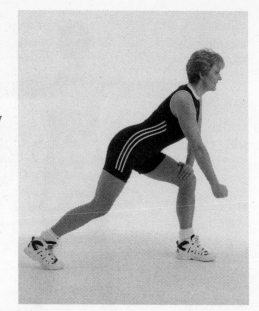

Squeeze your shoulder blades together and down and slowly bend elbow, raising it behind your body while sliding hand to hip. Repeat 12 times, then change legs and repeat with your left arm.
TIPS: Feel your shoulder blade squeeze towards your spine as you do the rows. In later weeks you can add a small weight to the working arm.

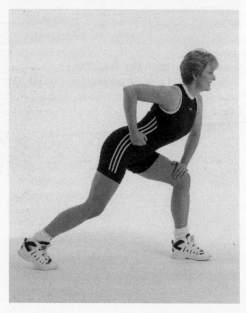

5 Bicep curls (for upper arm)
Stand in correct starting position with arms down and in front of you and palms away from you.

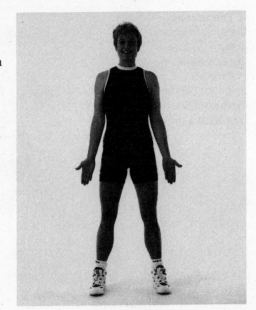

Bend elbows, keeping upper arms firmly into your body and lift hands towards shoulders. Slowly lower and repeat 12 times.
TIP: In later weeks, add hand weights, starting with 1kg (2lb) maximum each hand.

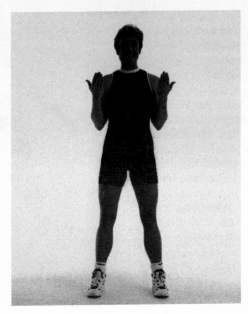

6 Tricep extensions (for backs of upper arms)
Stand in correct starting position with both arms bent and elbows pointing to back wall.

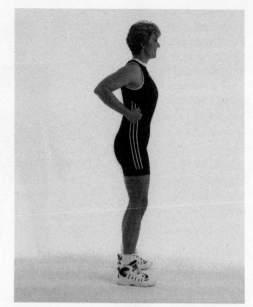

Now lengthen your arms out to the back. Return to start and repeat 12 times. **TIPS:** Feel the exercise working in the triceps. Keep upper arm still and parallel to the floor. Just move from the elbow. In later weeks add hand weights as above.

Now lie down on the floor for the rest of the exercises.

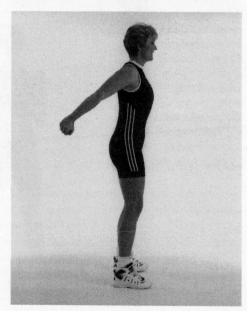

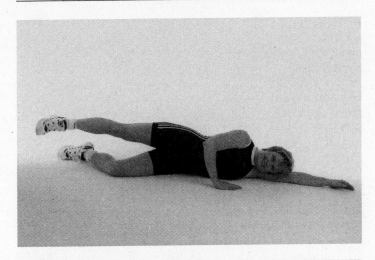

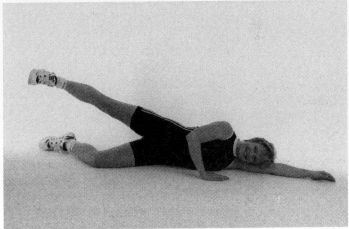

7 Side lying leg lifts (for outer thighs and hips)
Lie on your left side with your head resting on your arm and left leg
slightly bent. Now, keeping your body facing straight forward, top hip
directly over bottom hip, raise right leg slowly up, keeping knee and ankle
facing forward. Slowly lower and repeat 12 times.
TIPS: Don't turn your right leg up towards the ceiling as you do this
exercise, and keep your hips 'stacked'. Either of these movements will
decrease the effectiveness of the exercise.

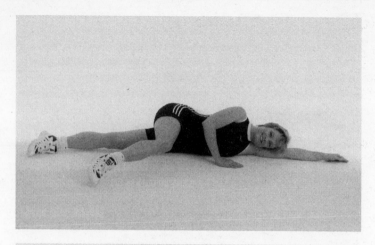

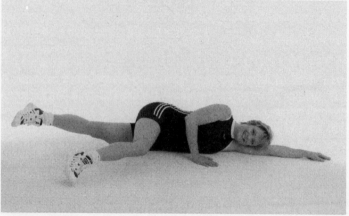

8 Side lying inner thigh lifts (for inner thighs)

Still lying on left side, straighten left leg and bring right leg over left leg in front of you with knee bent and elevated slightly off the floor. Now slowly raise left leg off the floor a few inches, or as far as you can, and slowly lower. Repeat 12 times.

TIP: Keep your hips at right angles to the floor. This isn't as easy as it looks; you may hardly be able to move your left leg up at all to begin with. Persevere!

Now turn over on to your right side and repeat exercises 7 and 8 on that side.

9 Press-ups (for chest, front shoulders, triceps)

Kneel on all fours with your knees directly under hips, fingers facing forward and hands slightly more than shoulder-width apart. Keeping your tummy pulled in and back lengthened, slowly lower your torso towards the floor by bending your elbows. When you have nearly reached the floor (or as far as you can go), slowly return to start and repeat 12 times.

TIPS: Do the movement slowly. Don't dip head in trying to reach the floor. In later weeks, to make the exercise harder, take your knees further back. Eventually you will be able to take your knees right back so the backs of your thighs make a straight line with your back.

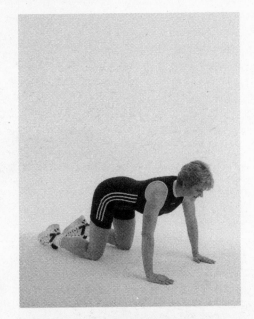

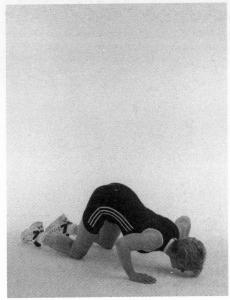

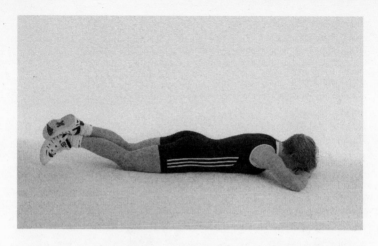

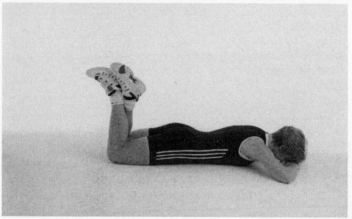

10 Prone hamstring curls (for backs of thighs)
Lie on your stomach with your arms bent and fingers under forehead,
arms flat on floor, legs stretched out behind you. Cross left ankle over
right ankle. Now slowly curl right lower leg in towards the back of your
right thigh, while pushing down with the left leg providing resistance,
curling in as far as you can. Feel your hamstring contract. Keep your hip
bones pressed on to the floor. Slowly return to start and repeat 12 times.
Repeat on the other leg.

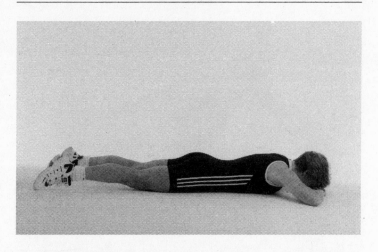

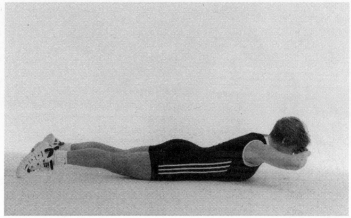

11 Back extensions (for lower back)
Lie on your stomach as above, keeping feet shoulder-width apart and legs lengthened, hip bones into floor. Slowly raise torso a couple of inches off the floor and return. Repeat 12 times.
TIP: Always keep your legs in contact with the floor.

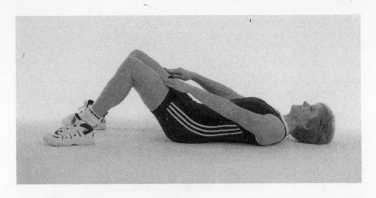

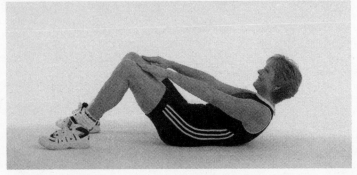

12 Curl-ups and pelvic floor tightener (for abdomen and pelvic floor)
Lie on your back with knees bent, feet flat on the floor. Tilt pelvis so your
tailbone points directly down from shoulders, bottom relaxed, and your
back is lightly touching the floor, arms at sides.

   Now concentrate on your abdominal area and on your pelvic floor (the
area around your vagina). Inhale, then tighten the pelvic floor muscles as if
trying to squeeze your vaginal entrance shut, and, as you do so, exhale and
pull your tummy in as you curl your torso up so your shoulder blades come
off the floor (if you can) and slide your hands up and forward towards knees.
Your lower back will flatten into the floor as you come up. Inhale as you
slowly lower, lengthening stomach muscles and relaxing pelvic floor.
Repeat 12 times.
TIPS: Don't allow lower back to hollow out as you lower your torso.
Concentrate on the effort coming from your abdomen, not your neck. In
later weeks you can take your shoulders a little further off the floor, and
to make the movement more difficult, you can place your fingers behind
your head, but don't pull your head with your hands.

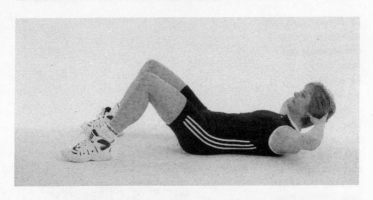

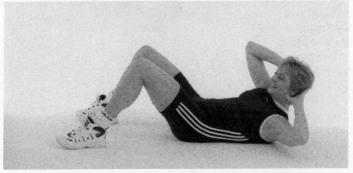

13 Diagonal curl-ups and pelvic floor tightener (for waist and pelvic floor)
Begin with your body in the start position as for previous exercise, but
this time have your hands lightly behind your head, elbows out.
Concentrating, again, on keeping those pelvic floor muscles tight, bring
right shoulder and upper back off floor, so that right shoulder moves
towards left knee. Slowly lower and repeat 12 times. Repeat on other
side.
TIPS: Don't bring your elbow in as you come up; this gives a false
impression that you are doing more work than you are. Keep the bent arm
in line with your raised shoulder; the effort should come from your
obliques (waist muscles). Exhale on the way up, inhale on the way down.
Don't forget to tighten those pelvic muscles before and during the
movement. A strong pelvic floor is good for your sex life and for helping
to prevent prolapse and stress incontinence in later life.

14 Reverse curls with pelvic floor tighteners (for abdomen and pelvic floor)
Lie on the floor as in previous two exercises, arms behind your head. Tighten pelvic floor area, cross ankles and bring knees up and over hips. Now, initiating the movement with the lower portion of your abdominal muscles, curl your hips in towards your ribs so that your hips lift slightly off the floor.

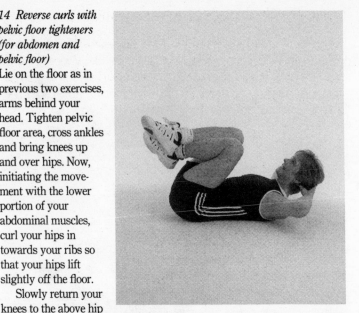

Slowly return your knees to the above hip position, then repeat 12 times. (Don't return feet to the floor until the set is finished, or you have done as many reverse curls as you can manage if you are currently doing less that that.)
TIP: This is a small curling movement. Don't try to get your hips further off the floor by bouncing or using your hands to push up. It's also easier to put your arms flat down by your sides with palms facing upwards.

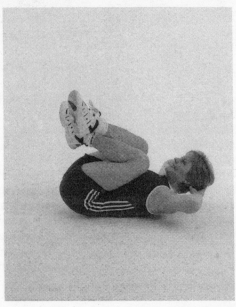

COOL-DOWN STRETCHES (3 minutes)

Hold each of these stretches for at least 10 seconds. Aim for more,
building up to 30 seconds as you get more flexible. Concentrate on
doing the stretches correctly and going into the movement more as
you relax. All these stretches are done lying or sitting on the floor.
Breathe calmly and deeply throughout.

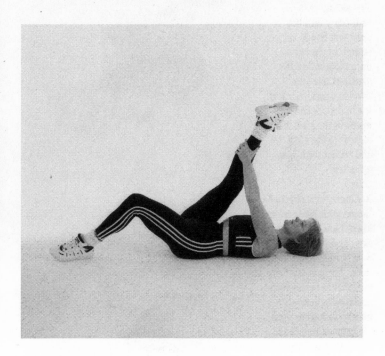

1 Hamstring stretch
Lie on your back with knees bent and feet flat on the floor. Bring the right
leg in (still bent) towards your chest then slowly lengthen the leg, clasping
your hands behind your right calf or back of thigh. Pull your leg in
towards your chest until you feel a stretch along the back of your thigh
(hamstring). Hold the stretch. Return to start and repeat with your left leg.
TIP: You may not be able to straighten your leg out during this stretch at
first but as the weeks go by you will be able to straighten it more. Try not
to push off from the foot that's on the floor. Keep the leg relaxed.

*2 Gluteal stretch
(bottom and hips)*
Lie on your back,
bend your knees with
your feet flat on the
floor. Cross your right
ankle over your left
thigh and bring your
legs slowly in
towards your chest
until you feel a
stretch in the right
buttock and hip. If
possible, use your
hands to pull your left
leg into your chest to
increase the stretch.
Return to the start
and repeat with your
other leg.

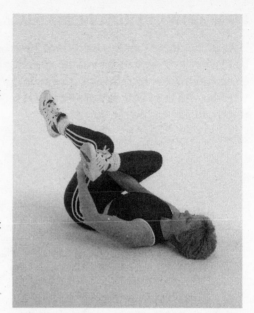

3 Lower back stretch
Lie on your back with
knees bent, feet on the
floor and lower back
lightly touching the
floor. Bring your
knees in towards your
chest, with your
hands clasped around
the back of your legs.
Use your hands to
pull your knees
gently as far in
towards your chest as
they will go. Feel the
stretch in your lower
back. Hold, slowly
release and return to
start.

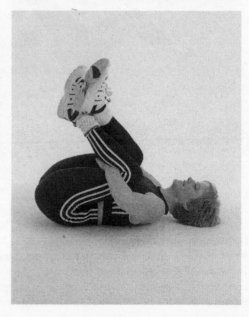

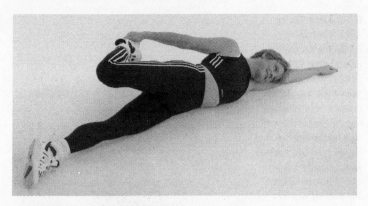

4 Quadriceps (front thigh) stretch
Turn on to your left side with left leg slightly bent and right hand
supporting your head. Flex your right knee and ankle and reach down to
hold your right foot with your right hand just below the ankle. Gently pull
your heel in towards your bottom, pushing hips backwards. Feel the
stretch down your right quadriceps. Hold, slowly return to start, turn over
and repeat with your left leg.

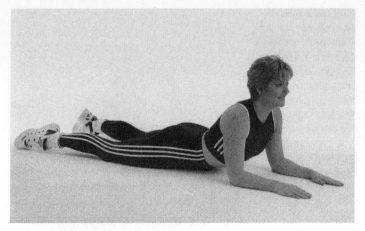

5 Abdominal stretch
Turn over and lie on your front. Bend your arms so that your elbows are
directly under your shoulders, your forearms flat on the floor and your
palms facing forward. Hold your upper body off the floor; lift your chest
and look forward; feel stretch along abdomen.

6 Abductor (outer thigh) stretch
Sit on the floor and extend your legs in front of you. Bend your right leg and cross it over your left leg, resting your right foot on the floor to the left of your left knee. Hug your bent leg into your chest. Hold the stretch, slowly release and repeat on the other side.

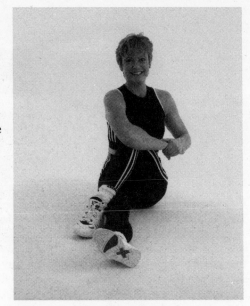

7 Adductor (inner thigh) stretch
Sit on the floor and bend your knees. Place the soles of your shoes together in front of you letting your legs fall to either side of your body. With your hands on the floor behind you, gently push each leg further towards the floor. Feel inner thigh stretch.
TIP: Keep the back long as if you are sitting against a wall, your chest lifted, shoulder-blades together and down.

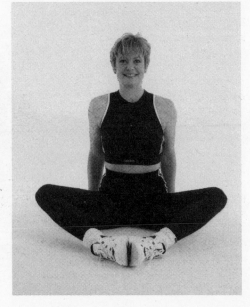

8 Chest stretch
Sit on the floor and place your hands behind your ears, with elbows out. Now press arms back and feel the stretch across your chest. Hold.

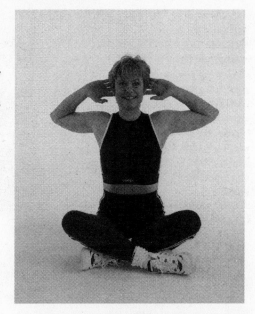

9 Shoulder stretch
Bring your right arm across your body, keeping your arm long but not locked. Use your left hand to press gently above your right elbow in towards your chest. Press your right shoulder down away from your ear for an even better stretch. Feel your right shoulder stretch. Hold, then slowly release and repeat on the other side.

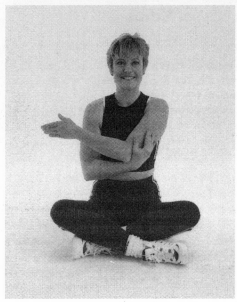

10 Side stretch
Sitting on the floor
with your legs
crossed and left arm
supporting you on the
floor, bring your right
arm up towards the
ceiling and over until
you feel the stretch up
your right side. Hold,
slowly return to start
and repeat on the
other side.

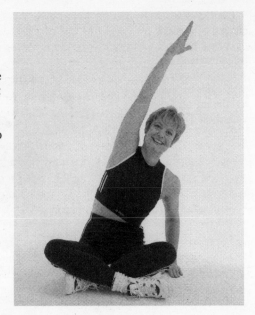

Optional Extras

Optional extra aerobics: see page 140.

Optional extra strength and tone: If you ticked many of the
boxes in the Section 2 symptoms analysis on page 131, you will
benefit from extra strength and toning work. The first thing to do
is master the basic routine as laid out on pages 153–166,
concentrating on building up to one good complete set of 12
repetitions of each exercise as described.

Once you have mastered one set, aim to build up to two sets of
each exercise. Or, if you have particularly weak areas which you
wish to build up – your stomach muscles are particularly poor, for
instance – you can concentrate simply on adding extra sets of the
low back and three stomach and waist exercises 11, 12, 13 and 14
(pages 163–6). Or, if your inner thighs seem particularly flabby,
you can concentrate on doing extra sets of exercise 8, the inner
thigh lifts on page 160.

It is *your* programme – you decide what work your body needs
most, and do extra on that.

Another option is to add one extra day a week of toning, making it four days a week instead of three. Only do this when you are used to exercise, and make sure your exercise sessions are spaced out evenly throughout the week.

Lastly, you could add on, or substitute, other tone and strength work, rather than the *Bodysense* 20-minute routine. Check down the Activities chart on pages 142–3. You will see all activities rated from one to three stars for upper body strength and for lower body strength. Choose any activity/ies that offer/s good strength benefits. You could mix and match, choosing one for lower body and one that's good for the upper body.

The point about exercising is that you shouldn't get bored, and this will offer you almost endless variety.

Optional extra stretch and relax: If you ticked many of the boxes in Sections 3 and 4 on page 132, you will benefit from adding on the four extra stretches that are described below *after* your cool-down stretches. You should also spend as long as you can on the cool-down stretches themselves.

1 Spinal stretch (for spine and neck)
Sit on the floor with your legs crossed and clasp your fingers gently across the back of your head, letting your head drop forward. Stay upright and let the weight of your arms stretch your neck and top of spine. Keep holding your head gently through the stretch. To further the spine stretch you can also round the back into a curl towards your lap. Stretch for one minute.

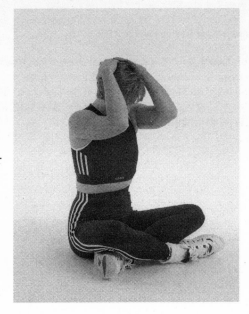

2 Shoulder stretch (for upper back and shoulders)
Sitting as in previous stretch, lift arms and clasp hands in front of you
with palms facing outwards. Push your hands forward as you round your
back into the stretch. Feel the stretch in the back of your shoulders and
upper back. Hold for 30 seconds or more.

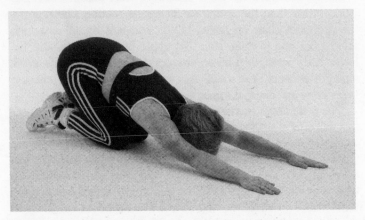

3 Back and shoulder stretch (for back, upper arms, chest)
Kneel on the floor, sitting back on your heels, and slide your hands across
the floor in front of you until your forehead nearly touches the floor and
your back is stretched out. Hold for 30 seconds or more. (See above.)

4 Long body stretch (for stomach, chest, waist, underarms and relaxation)
Lie on your back on the floor with your legs out straight. Lift your arms
above your head until they rest on the floor. Feel your whole body
stretching out. Concentrate on one part after another – first feel your
waist elongating and your abdomen stretching. Then, as you relax the
stretch, feel your arms sinking further into the floor and your lower back
releasing. Lengthen the body again and hold the stretch for 30 seconds
then let it go. Relax for 30 seconds then do the full stretch again. Finally,
relax for a minute and sit up gradually.

Optional extra pelvic, stomach and lower back release: If
you ticked section five on page 132, you will benefit from adding
these extra exercises on to the end of your basic strength and tone
routine during Phase Three (just before your period and during
the first two days of your period). These will take you only 2–3
minutes to do.

1 Abdomen and hip rotations

Stand in the correct starting position. Now sway your hips gently from side to side ten times, then forward and back ten times and finally in a clockwise circle 10 times, then an anti-clockwise circle 10 times. Concentrate on keeping the rest of your body still as your hips move.

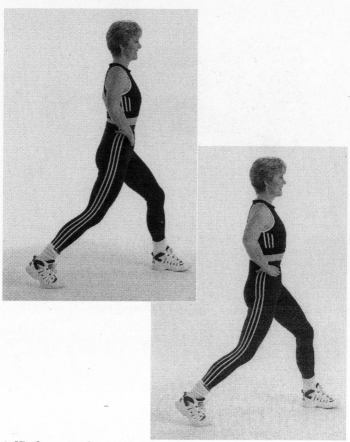

2 Hip flexor stretch

Stand with your arms by your sides, feet hip-width apart. Now bring your right leg forward, bent at knee, and take your left leg back into a lunge position with your back heel off the floor. Push your back thigh (tailbone) forward and the top of your pelvis backwards. Return to the start and repeat with your left leg to the front. (See above.)

3 Lower back release
Repeat Stretch 3 from Cool-down stretches (page 168). Now, in the same
starting position, hold on to your knees and rotate your legs in a gentle
clockwise circle 10 times. Rotate anti-clockwise 10 times.

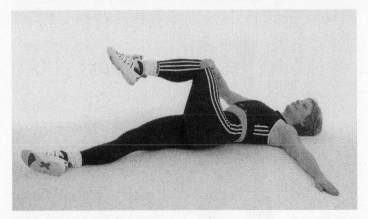

4 Hip release
Lie on your back with your left leg straight, right leg bent and in towards
your chest. Now, take your right leg across your body, keeping your knee
bent at a 90° angle, using your left hand to help bring your leg across, on
the outside of the leg. Keep your opposite leg straight. (See above.)

Optional extra body alignment exercises: If you ticked
many of the boxes in section 6 on page 132, you suffer from poor
body alignment and posture and will benefit from doing the
following exercises which will take you 2–3 minutes. The first
three can be done every day – the last one can be done three times
a week with your strength and tone exercises. You will also
benefit from doing extra sets of the low back and abdominal
exercises – 11, 12, 13 and 14 in the basic routine.

1 Pelvic tilt
Wearing a leotard or underwear only, stand sideways on to a full-length
mirror. Keep your ribcage lifted and still. Keep your bottom muscles
relaxed as you rock your pelvis so that your tailbone points forward and
your back is flat (tummy muscles should be controlling this movement
with no tension in the buttocks). Then rock your pelvis so that your
tailbone points backwards and your back slightly arches. Rock back and

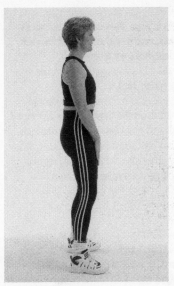

Incorrect posture

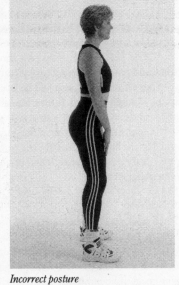

Incorrect posture

forth between these two extreme points several times to derive pelvic awareness. Now settle into a position between these two extremes where the tailbone points directly to the floor. You have your *natural* curve in your lower back, tummy muscles slightly tense, bottom relaxed. This position is called Neutral Pelvis.

Now squeeze your shoulder blades together and down, and pull your head back so that the ears line up with the shoulders. All of the natural curves of your spine should be apparent. This position is called the Neutral Spine.

Right: *Correct posture known as Neutral Spine demonstrating the natural curves of our spine. This position is the safest position for our spine to be in, day in, day out.*

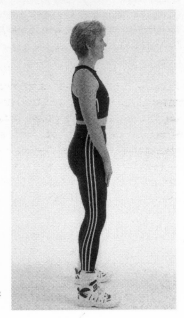

2 *Front posture check*

Stand face on to the mirror now and check your stance. Your shoulders should be relaxed and sloping to the same degree either side. Your neck should be long and there shouldn't be deep hollows above your collarbone. If there are, bring your shoulder blades together towards your spine and practise exercise 4 frequently (page 156).

Your waist and hips should be level either side. Your knees should be facing straight forward. If they face inward, do the pelvic tilt as described above and concentrate on using your gluteal muscles to bring your legs into alignment. Do extra outer and inner thigh work (see exercises 1, 2, 7 and 8 in the basic routine). If your foot arches are flattened out, regular lower body strength, stretch and re-alignment exercises will help to correct this problem.

3 *Wall test*

Stand with your back against a flat wall. Can you stand so that your bottom, shoulder blades and back of head all touch the wall at the same time? Practise this stance. When you have it, walk a step or two forward from the wall and practise walking around the room in the same alignment. If you find this very difficult, don't worry – time, patience and the basic exercises and stretches plus this section will help you to correct the alignment. The pelvic awareness, abdominal and back exercises (especially exercises 11 and 12) and the following exercise will help most.

4 Stooped shoulder correction

Kneel down on a mat or cushion and place one foot forward. Rest your chest on your front knee, keeping your back lengthened and your head and neck in line with your spine (i.e., neck long, ears over shoulders). Arms placed down by your front foot with thumbs pointing inward. Squeeze your shoulder blades together and down as you bend your elbows and draw them up and behind you. Keep your hands as far away from your body as possible.

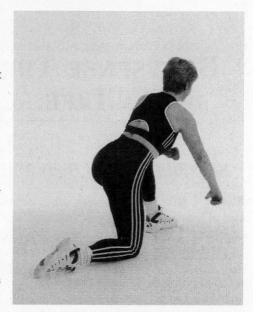

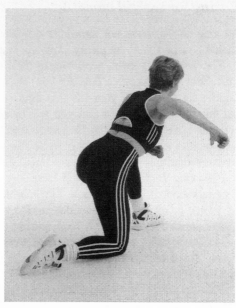

8

BODYSENSE THROUGH LIFE

· Sensible Ways to Body Maintenance ·

When you have reached a reasonable weight and shape, and a level of fitness with which you are happy (and please, let me say again what I said in Chapter One – that a 'reasonable' weight is not the same as being thin, and that a 'reasonable' shape is not the same as a perfect one) you need to know what you should do to maintain your body in its optimum state.

Eating for weight control

As long as you have not aimed for too low a bodyweight, you should now be able to eat plenty while maintaining your new size.

The 'average' woman, according to the Department of Health, eats about 1940 calories a day. As you won't want to be counting calories for the rest of your life this figure doesn't really matter, but what I can tell you is that you will be able to eat *more* than you did while following the *Bodysense* diet, and, if you keep up with regular exercise, you may even be able to eat *more* than that 'average' figure.

Following *Bodysense* you will have lost weight slowly on a generous amount of food. Phase Three, which you will probably have been following for at least one week a month, contains about 1,600 calories a day of healthy food, so now, in order to begin your maintenance programme, all you need to do is begin following Phase Three on a more permanent basis, but increasing your portions at every meal by approximately 20%.

Then to keep your body healthy and your weight more or less constant, simply follow the eating advice in Chapter Three.

To sum up:

- Eat evenly spaced out meals to avoid hunger.
- Eat plenty of the low GI foods (see page 43) to avoid hunger.
- As well as three meals, have two snacks a day based on the 'best mix' ideas on page 58.
- Remember that your body's needs will vary at different times. When your appetite is small, eat small portions (but don't skip meals). When your appetite is bigger, eat bigger portions and fill up on low GI foods.
- Remember to listen to your body and read the signals it gives out.
- Pre-menstruation, always eat Phase Three types of meals and avoid alcohol, simple carbohydrates and high-salt foods.
- Don't go too low on fat, especially unsaturated fats which women need in small quantities for good health. Eat enough of the pure vegetable oils, especially olive oil and corn oil. Eat some nuts, seeds, oily vegetables and oily fish.
- Think of food as enjoyable body fuel – keep it in perspective.

An alternative
As an alternative to increasing your portion sizes, you could include an extra best-mix snack into your body's eating – so you have three meals and three best-mix snacks.

This option is ideal for women who prefer snacking and/or who have a long day. For example, if you get up at 6.30am and go to bed at midnight, you may find an extra, substantial snack is just what you need late evening to prevent hunger pangs. Or, if you have early lunch and a late supper, you may like the safety net of two snacks instead of one between lunchtime and supper.

Before your period, in the typical Phase Three time of the month, this may be the preferred way of eating.

The food charts
As a general rule, it shouldn't be necessary for you to count calories in order to control your weight. Eating the right types of foods in the right balance and at the right times, as you have learnt in the earlier chapters, is a much more realistic approach. But sometimes you may want to find out the calorie content of a

new food, or devise your own recipes. You may want to see if a particular food fits in with the ideal pattern of *plenty* of carbohydrate, a *little* fat and *enough* protein.

Then you can look up the food charts in Appendix One. The notes preceding the charts will give you more information on how to use them.

Beating those food addictions

Most women who report problems with food 'addictions' say that their main problem is chocolate. So I'm going to talk about chocolate for a bit – but when I say 'chocolate', if your particular passion has always been gooey cakes, or biscuits, or crisps, or any other food that your body can well do without quite happily but that you have always felt the need for, then think of that food when I say 'chocolate'. The advice is pertinent through the whole range of typical 'addiction' foods.

Chocolate cravings – when you suddenly think of chocolate even when you aren't near any, and badly wish you had some – are usually because your blood sugar level is low (see page 45). This is a physical craving and is brought about because you haven't been following the *Bodysense* Eating Plan properly. If you eat regular meals with plenty of low GI foods, plenty of fibre, a little protein and fat, and you quite religiously stick to your two extra 'best-mix' type snacks between meals, then your blood sugar levels should not dip so low that you begin to crave something sweet.

If you are grabbed by a strong craving for a sweet food and it is too late for me to say, 'Ah, but you should have . . .' then the answer is to eat a best-mix snack. This will satisfy you and stop the 'rebound' effect that a high-sugar snack would bring – make you crave more before too long.

The other type of chocolate problem is when you have some – this may not be your own doing, someone may have given you a box of chocs, for instance – and once you have begun to eat it, you can't stop. This is usually because chocolate feels fantastic in the mouth, it glides easily and quickly down your throat and is, simply, a pleasurable oral experience.

Now if this is only likely to happen to you at Christmas,

birthdays and Easter – then quite honestly, I wouldn't worry about it! Even eating a whole 1lb box of chocolates will only put just over half a pound of fat on you at the most. Phase One eating for a few days afterwards will redress the balance.

The point is that I don't think you should live without every last wicked indulgence for the rest of your life. But the interesting thing is that if you have been for several weeks (for example) *without* any chocolate, you may well find (probably will find) that you no longer have the taste for it; try as you might to eat that box of chocolates, you will find it impossible.

Bodysense truly has retrained your tastebuds!

The thing about chocolate is to stop feeling completely guilty for liking it, or the idea of it, at least. Tell yourself you can have a bit now and then when you want to. Don't tell yourself 'never again'.

The only rule is – don't eat it when you are hungry. Eat it after a meal or a best-mix snack.

Alcohol

Women are drinking more alcohol than ever and if you drink more than a couple of bottles of wine a week (or equivalent), obviously it will be harder for you to maintain your weight as you are adding calories to your diet that you don't really notice. Alcohol, like sugar, contains little or no nutrients and, although red wine may help to protect against heart disease, there really is little to justify recommending that you drink more than a glass or two of wine with your main meal.

If you do drink, and you want to avoid putting on weight, you will have to be meticulous about cutting back on equivalent types of food in your diet – the sugar-based things like sweets, sugar, glucose drinks, and so on, that also provide little or no nutrients except calories. And you will have to pay very special attention to getting maximum nutrition in your meals.

Alcohol is one of the pleasures of life for many of us – but for your body's sake, don't let it become *too* much of a pleasure. There are other ways of relaxing – exercise, music, a hot bath and a book, sex, a good video.

If you use alcohol to help you dismiss your inhibitions (the other main reason we drink) then take some time to think why you need to do this. See if you can alter your lifestyle, your friends, or whatever, so that you no longer need to find false courage. And think about the fact that, sometimes, a certain amount of self-control is a good thing!

Exercise and Body Maintenance

If you have read Chapter Six, and been following the exercise programme in Chapter Seven, then you don't really need me to tell you that your body thrives on movement and activity.

It is obvious, then, that the exercise shouldn't stop just because you have reached the shape/size and/or fitness level that you wanted to achieve.

It takes only approximately three months for your fit and well-toned body to revert to being out of tone and unfit. But to maintain the levels you have achieved can be done in around two hours a week.

What to do

Fit three aerobic sessions a week into your life, preferably of 30 minutes each, but 20 will do at a pinch. The more vigorous you can make these sessions, the more benefit you will get from them in the short space of time, (for example, a 20-minute jog or uphill cycle ride will do more for your fitness than a 20-minute fairly easy walk).

Then fit at least two strength, tone and stretch sessions into your week, spaced evenly.

This could be an advanced stage of the programme in Chapter Seven, or you could try something different if you are confident – a class, a gym circuit, a video – it is up to you. The one thing you don't want to do with your strength, tone and stretch is to get bored.

Keep your routines interesting and keep your motivation high by reminding yourself of all the benefits you are giving your body.

(If you exercise in a particular room, you could write out the benefits that appear on a sheet of paper and pin it on the wall.)

Plan your session times at the beginning of the week and write them in your diary. Rope in a friend to do your sessions with you – less chance then that you will opt out at the last minute.

And use the activities chart on pages 142–3 to find new sports and activities to help you to keep moving.

There will come a point for almost all of us when we can't get any fitter – because to do so would involve more time than we genuinely can make available. That is the time to be content with the fitness and the shape you have, or to find new ways to make the work that you do even harder. But there will still come a point when you can't make it harder either.

That doesn't matter. The fact is that you have been kind to your body by making it as fit as possible. Now keeping it that way is more important than anything else you can do for it.

Extras
If you have been doing any of the optional extra exercise sequences – for posture, relaxation, and so on, you can continue with these. Twice a week is ideal, added on to your strength, tone and stretch routine.

If you give up these extras you may find your original problem will return. It may not. It could be that the basic routine is enough to keep the initial problem at bay. But it isn't really worth taking the risk of finding out.

Exercise and weight maintenance

Lastly, if you have previously had problems in maintaining your weight even though you don't think you eat a great deal, I can't stress enough the importance of exercise to you.

Exercise will help you to maintain your new weight for life in three ways:

- Aerobic exercise burns up the calories that provide the fuel that your body needs to do the work involved.
- Strength exercise builds or maintains muscle mass which is more metabolically active than any other body matter – in other words, the more lean tissue (muscle) in your body, the more calories it will burn.

● Exercise, in conjunction with the right diet, can help to control your appetite. If you can't believe this, try the test for yourself: Next time you are feeling a little hungry, do a 15-minute walk or gentle workout and at the end of it, your need for food will have disappeared.

· *Bodysense in Pregnancy* ·

When you are pregnant, both for your own sake and that of your baby, you need to eat *healthily*, you need to eat *enough* and you need to stay fit.

Bodysense offers everyone the chance to do exactly that, of course – but throughout pregnancy both your food and fitness needs are slightly different from other times in your life, so in this section we'll look at the adaptations you need to make to the basic programme for your optimum well-being during those important months.

Pregnancy and your weight

Your view about your weight during your pregnancy will probably fall into one of two categories: either you will do all you can to ensure that you put on as little weight as possible and you'll knock yourself out to be back to your pre-pregnancy figure within weeks of the birth; or you will look upon pregnancy as a wonderful time to indulge yourself, eat for two – and be happy to go along with the idea that a several stone weight gain is natural, not unhealthy.

The most natural – and sensible – view is somewhere between those two extremes. But the exact way you eat during your pregnancy will depend to a great extent upon what size you are when you first discover you are pregnant.

If you are overweight at the start of pregnancy: The least sensible idea – and one of the most dangerous for your growing baby, especially in its first few months in your womb – is to embark on a crash diet. If you don't eat enough throughout your pregnancy, you risk having a low birth weight baby which greatly increases his or her risk of death, infections, and other disorders.

The latest recommendations (from an official Board in the USA) suggest that overweight women should simply adapt their calorie intake slightly so that they gain less weight by the end of the pregnancy than average weight or thin women.

Very obese women (several stones overweight at the start of pregnancy) should aim to gain least weight of all.

You can use your Body Mass Index to help you to decide whether you need to gain less weight than average during your pregnancy. (If you've forgotten your BMI, see page 13 in Chapter One.)

If your BMI (at start of pregnancy) is between 26 and 29, you are classed as mildly to moderately overweight and the recommendation is that you gain between 7kg (14lbs) and 11kgs (22lbs). The higher your BMI between those two levels, the nearer to that 7kg level you should aim for.

If your BMI (at start of pregnancy) is 30 or over you are classed as very overweight (obese) and the recommendation is that you gain 6kg (12lbs) but no less than that.

The best way to achieve these lower weight gain levels is by following the weight maintenance advice. This suggests that you eat around 1,940 calories a day along *Bodysense* lines and should certainly be appropriate for the first six months of pregnancy, in terms of energy (calories).

Then, for the last three months, you should add on a few extra calories – about 200 a day, which you can achieve either by increasing portions slightly or by adding on a 200-calorie healthy snack such as a best-mix snack.

If your ante-natal clinic doctor or dietician feels you are gaining weight either too slowly or too quickly, you can adjust the amount you eat a little either way.

You should also follow the special nutrition guidelines for pregnancy that appear later in this section.

If you are overweight and pregnant, it *is* important to control your weight gain and not pile on stones and stones because, just as too few calories can be bad for you and the baby, a huge weight gain during pregnancy (or carrying many surplus stones right from the start of the pregnancy) can be just as risky. High weight gain is associated with more pregnancy complications, longer labour – and the likelihood of remaining obese after the baby is born.

If you are not overweight at the start of the pregnancy: If your BMI is between 20 and 25 (average weight) then you should aim to put on between 11.5kg (23lbs) and 16kg (32lbs).

Interestingly, to achieve such levels of weight gain, the official UK recommendations are that pregnant women of average weight increase their food intake by a mere 200 calories a day for the last three months of the pregnancy only. Thin women (BMI under 20) may need to eat more to put on the 12.5kg (25lbs) to 18kg (36lbs) that is recommended for them.

One reason for this low extra food intake in order to gain the required weight in pregnancy is thought to be that pregnant women use less energy (they move more slowly, sit and rest for longer periods, etc.). Another explanation could be that the pregnant body lowers its metabolic rate.

Whatever the reason, you don't need to 'eat for two' throughout your pregnancy. Again, it helps to listen to your body and read its signals. If you feel genuinely hungry, eat. Eat the *Bodysense* way and you will know that you are giving your baby a healthy diet as well as yourself – but you must follow the special nutrition guidelines for pregnancy below to ensure you get enough of the vitamins and minerals that you need when you are pregnant.

I suggest that if your BMI is between 20 and 25, you use the weight maintenance guidelines earlier in this chapter for the first six months of your pregnancy and then add on around 200 calories a day of good, healthy food in the last three months. If your weight gain is slower than average, eat a little more, if you find you are piling weight on too fast, cut down a little.

Don't forget your ante-natal clinic dietician is there to help you if there is anything connected with your eating plan you're not sure about.

Special nutrition guidelines for pregnancy

All pregnant women should ensure they consume adequate amounts of various vitamins and minerals right from the early stages of pregnancy. The following is a list of the nutrients you have a special extra need for during pregnancy with some examples of the best sources. Within the *Bodysense* programme, make sure you choose plenty of those foods.

Folic acid   (Your ante-natal clinic will supply you with a folic acid supplement which you should take.) Yeast extract (Marmite), pulses, wheatgerm, brewer's yeast, dark green vegetables, nuts.

Vitamin B group   As folic acid, also whole grains, (e.g., brown rice, wholewheat pasta), eggs, fish, cheeses.

Vitamin C   Fresh fruits, saladstuffs and vegetables*, especially red peppers, blackcurrants, parsley, broccoli, Brussels sprouts, cabbage, strawberries, spinach, oranges, grapefruit.

Vitamin D   Main sources are eggs and oily fish. Or exposure to sunlight when Vitamin D is synthesised by the body. Supplements may be provided by your ante-natal clinic if necessary.

Calcium   You need plenty of calcium for your baby's rapidly growing bones. It appears that your own bone density diminishes slightly during the first three months of pregnancy in order to provide a calcium 'reservoir'. Also, your body absorbs more calcium from the food you eat – so in theory you may not need any more calcium than before you were pregnant – but I wouldn't take any chances and the extra 500mg a day recommended in the USA sounds sensible to me! Eat plenty of low-fat dairy produce such as skimmed milk and yogurt, plus leafy green vegetables, fish, eggs, pulses, broad beans, and dried apricots.

Iron   If you had a tendency to anaemia before your pregnancy you may be prescribed iron tablets (which sometimes make you constipated) so it is wise to ensure you get enough in your diet by eating plenty of: pulses, wheatgerm, seeds, egg yolk, leafy green vegetables, dried apricots and peaches, very lean red meat, wholemeal flour, oats, nuts, tofu and bulgar wheat.

When you are pregnant you should also watch your intake of certain things that could be harmful, such as:

Alcohol   It's advisable to give up alcohol altogether before conception and during pregnancy. If you do drink, make it an occasional glass of wine at most. Heavy drinking is linked with

*Stored in cool, dark conditions and eaten as fresh as possible.

low birth weight and various abnormalities in the baby, as is smoking.

Liver and liver products These contain very high amounts of vitamin A (retinol) which, in excessive doses, is toxic to the unborn baby.

Vitamin A supplements If you are trying to conceive, the Department of Health recommends that you do not use vitamin A supplements or fish liver oil capsules. During pregnancy, these supplements can be taken as long as they contain only up to 1,250ug of vitamin A per dose.

To sum up
Eat a varied diet containing plenty of the vitamin and mineral-rich foods (except liver) and eat enough to put on your optimum amount of weight.

The *Bodysense* system contains all the right kinds of foods for pregnancy and its maintenance system can be followed through pregnancy if you bear the above extra recommendations in mind.

After the birth
You can begin the *Bodysense* maintenance diet or, if you need to lose weight, the Phase Three eating plan with 250ml ($1/2$ pint) a day extra skimmed milk. If breastfeeding, and/or you are losing weight at more than 1lb per week, you may need to eat more than this. Increase portions until weight loss slows down.

Breastfeeding, by the way, uses up at least 500 calories of energy a day from your body so it is a great way to return to your pre-pregnancy size without having to cut down on calories.

Exercise during pregnancy

How hard you exercise during your pregnancy depends firstly upon how much exercise you did before you became pregnant. If you have been used to, say, the *Bodysense* programme of exercise, including strength and tone work, stretching and aerobics, then you will be able to continue with this, in all probability, at least for the first few months.

If you go into your pregnancy without having exercised recently, it is unwise to try to begin any new régime.

Either way, you should always check with your clinic or doctor and tell them what exercise you are doing. The following are simple guidelines:

● Exercise regularly for short periods of time.
● Avoid exercising in hot conditions.
● Exercise to a 'comfortable' level – up to level 6 on the perceived effort table (see page 138).
● If you are feeling ill or tired, don't exercise.
● If you have a history of or likelihood of miscarriage, don't exercise in the first few months of pregnancy.
● If you have any bleeding, don't exercise.
● If you have any medical condition, e.g., heart disease or diabetes, don't exercise.
● Listen to your body signals – if a move or any exercise doesn't feel 'right', don't do it.
● Avoid lifting weights.
● Avoid high-impact aerobic exercise (e.g., jogging, advanced aerobics classes) which can cause long-term joint problems (see notes about the hormone relaxin below).

Special points and tips

● As your 'bump' gets bigger, you will want to stop doing any exercise that involves lying on your tummy, and many women can't lie flat on their backs to exercise in the last month or two. Stop doing any exercise that feels uncomfortable.

It sounds like a contradiction in terms to offer any kind of abdominal toning exercise at this stage, but you can keep those poor stretched 'abs' in marginal trim by kneeling on all-fours and rounding out your back as you gently but firmly pull your abdominal area up towards your back.

● *Stretching*. You will enjoy stretching your legs, your arms, your shoulders and your chest during your pregnancy but it is advisable not to do extra stretch work on your upper, mid and lower back. This is because when you are pregnant your body naturally produces a hormone – relaxin – that softens your pelvis in preparation for the birth – and also softens other joints in your body, including your spine. Extra stretching may make the effects of this worse and result in backache, and may weaken the back long term. Concentrate on keeping your back strong, instead, which will help your posture throughout pregnancy and help you to carry the baby, especially in the last few weeks.

● Learning the correct breathing technique is an important exercise for later in your pregnancy. This will also help you to relax. Your ante-natal clinic will give you breathing exercises and it's always a good idea to go to ante-natal classes for more advice on breathing and exercise, too.

After the birth

You can gradually get back to your pre-pregnancy routines. If you are new to exercise, now is a very motivational time to start. You can begin gentle curl-ups for that flabby tum within days of the birth! And a daily walk will do you good.

To sum up:

If you keep as fit as your pregnancy allows, you will probably have an easier and more enjoyable pregnancy than if you do nothing. The increased stamina, muscle strength and energy that comes through exercise – in fact, all the benefits you learnt about in Chapter Six, are likely to help your body through what is, after all, a very demanding time for it. You will also help to prevent pregnancy problems such as varicose veins, backache and leg cramps.

If you would like more information on exercise during pregnancy, I recommend *Fit for Birth* by Lucy Jackson (Thorsons £8.99).

· *Bodysense in the Menopause* · *and After*

When your menopause begins – usually between the ages of 45 and 55 – your periods will become less and less regular until, after a year or two, they stop altogether. And the level of the main female hormone, oestrogen, in the body drops considerably.

Research had indicated that around 60 per cent of women have no symptoms or only mild symptoms of the menopause (such as hot flushes or headaches), so the majority of us will go through this year or two as normal – and carry on afterwards as normal.

However, a wise approach to nutrition, weight control and exercise during and after the menopause can have a real effect on the quality of life during this time, so in this section we will look at these areas and suggest adaptations that you can make if you are approaching, or in, your menopause.

Weight control and the menopause

After the age of 25 or so, the rate at which our bodies burn up calories (our metabolic rate) gradually slows down. We need to consume around 50 fewer calories a day for every five years older than 25 we are. So, for instance, by the time you are 50 you will need to eat about 200 calories a day less than you did at 30 to maintain the same weight.

This may largely be explained by the natural reduction in lean tissue in our bodies as we get older. Our lean tissue (muscle) is more metabolically active than any other body matter. Also, we become less active the older we get, and activity burns up calories.

During and after the menopause, any surplus fat that we do put on settles on our stomachs and waists. This is probably because after menopause our bodies contain more of the male hormone, testosterone, and central fat distribution (the 'apple shape') is more of a male characteristic than a female one.

This tendency to put on weight as we get older, even if we don't eat any more than we used to, is not entirely a bad thing. Indeed, I would say it is healthier for you to weigh up to a stone more than you did when young, if you were slim then. That is because the thinner you are, the more at risk you are of developing osteoporosis, the disease that reduces your bone mass and can cause skeletal and posture problems and bone fractures in later years.

Also, women around the menopausal years who carry more body fat also carry more oestrogen, which in turn helps to prevent or minimise osteoporosis and can act on the body in almost the same way as hormone replacement therapy (HRT).

Bigger women have stronger bones! And as osteoporosis is one of *the* major miseries of old age, occurring to a greater or lesser degree in most women, it makes sense now, even more than before, to aim for a reasonable weight bearing your age in mind, rather than a too-slim weight.

That is not to say you should be, or need to be, fat.

You can follow the complete *Bodysense* diet, choosing which phase to use at any given time by following the tips on pages 46–49, if you need to lose weight. Try to stick to Phase Two for at least half of the time, slot in the odd Phase One day, and save Phase Three days for when you feel the need to eat a bit more, and you should lose weight steadily – though don't expect fast losses. If you can lose even ½–1lb (225–500g) a week, that is equivalent to 2–4 (12–24kg) stone a year, which seems fine to me!

When slimming, it is important that you build activity into your life, to help to burn up the calories (see below).

If you don't need to lose weight, simply follow the weight maintenance plan tips at the beginning of this chapter.

Whether slimming or not, you should also bear in mind the special nutritional tips for women in their menopause which are listed below.

The menopause and special nutritional needs

Increased need for calcium   Throughout your life it is important to consume enough calcium to build strong bones. Until you are about 35, your bone mass increases so calcium intake during these formative years is vital. Then, gradually, bone mass begins to decrease, at a very slow rate (of about half to one per cent a year) until the age of 50.

Between the ages of 50 and 60 (or the menopausal years and the few years afterwards) bone loss in women accelerates and up to five per cent of bone mass is lost on average *every year*! One way to help to slow down this bone loss is to consume more calcium – at least 1,500mg a day, either from food or with calcium supplements, because during menopause our bodies absorb calcium less easily.

Here are the best sources of calcium in the diet, with amounts in mg per 100g (3½ oz) of product:

Parmesan cheese	1,200	Prawns	150
Seaweed	1,000	Chick peas	140
Cheddar cheese	800	Kidney beans	140
Edam cheese	740	Egg yolk	130
Molasses	684	Milk, all kinds	120
Sardines (including bone)	550	Muesli	120
Tofu	530	Black-eye beans	110
Feta or Camembert cheese	380	Broad beans	104
Pilchards	300	Broccoli	100
Dried figs	280	Rhubarb	100
Almonds	250	Soft cheese	98
Kale	250	Currants	95
Soya beans	225	Salmon	93
Mussels	200	Spinach	93
Brazil nuts	180	Dried apricots	92
Yogurt	180	Spring greens	86
Haricot beans	180	Butter beans	85
Chinese leaves	154	Savoy cabbage	75

Fortunately, many of the richest calcium-giving foods are also the ones that contain plenty of other nutritional 'goodies' such as other vitamins and minerals, fibre and protein, and thus feature prominently in the *Bodysense* diet.

Other nutritional factors affecting bone loss: You should make sure that you don't consume excessive amounts of *protein* or *salt*, because both can prevent calcium absorption. It's wise to keep salt intake low, anyway, for other health reasons and the *Bodysense* diet does this, as well as offering sensible quantities of protein.

You should also limit your intake of *alcohol* which may contribute to excessive bone loss. It's wise to do so, anyway, for your general health.

As we've already seen, *low body weight* contributes to osteoporosis, *smoking* has been linked with rapid bone loss, too. Lastly, a high *caffeine* intake (found in tea, coffee, colas and chocolate) has also been linked with increased bone loss but this isn't proven.

Increased need for fibre: Forty per cent of mid-life women suffer from diverticular disease (irritable bowel) and 25% of people over

50 have haemorrhoids (piles). Both of these problems can be minimised by increasing the fibre in your diet to keep your digestive system and bowels regular.

The best sources of fibre are: all pulses and lentils, fresh and dried fruits, vegetables, whole grains and All-Bran breakfast cereal.

Again, all these foods appear in the *Bodysense* diet but, as it is usually up to you to choose your selection of fruit and vegetables, make sure you have plenty of variety and large portions.

Menopause and exercise

Exercise is important throughout your life, as we've seen in Chapter Six – and the menopause is no exception.

Research shows that if you do no exercise at all (e.g., if you are in bed ill) after only a few days, there is a measurable reduction in your calcium levels, and if you were to stay in bed for only a few weeks, there is a measurable reduction in bone density.

Conversely, regular (though not excessive) exercise of the weight-bearing kind (e.g., walking) can *increase* bone density. Even if you are in your menopause or beyond it, regular weight-bearing activity can slow down the rate of bone loss – and can also help to prevent fractures by improving your muscle tone and balance.

So in the fight against osteoporosis, exercise is a must.

Here are some of the other reasons why you will benefit from doing some regular exercise throughout the menopause and afterwards:

- Exercise burns calories so will help you to keep your weight under control, at a time when many women find they are putting weight on.
- Exercise helps to prevent constipation, a complaint common to many women at this time.
- Exercise will help you to feel good about yourself at a time when some women feel a sense of regret at the passing of their child-bearing years.
- Exercise will help your muscles to stay strong – i.e., keep their bulk. Under-used muscles lose bulk and strength at a rate of up to 2kg (5lbs) every decade.

What exercise?

You can follow the plan in Chapter Seven because it is suitable for all ages and abilities. But remember:

- If you are not used to exercise, start gently. Try – but don't overstrain. Muscles, ligaments, tendons, and so on that haven't been used for years are more at risk of injury.
- Don't compare yourself with other people. Fitness can increase quickly in older people so it's well worth carrying on.
- Remember to do weight-bearing exercise for your bones. Weight bearing aerobic exercise includes (for lower body): walking, tennis, golf, basketball, aerobics, Step. For upper body: rowing, tennis. And many of the exercises in the strength and tone plan in Chapter Seven involve bearing some of your own bodyweight (e.g., the press-ups) so will help to increase bone density.

Remember, *Bodysense* is about having the right attitude to your body and being kind to it throughout life. With the right food, the right exercise, and the right approach, you and your body can live happily together whatever your age or circumstances. Don't let that go!

Apply *Bodysense* – for life!

Appendix I

FOOD CHARTS

Use the charts that follow to help you to devise a well balanced maintenance diet. Here are some notes to help you:

Remember that a healthy diet – that will also help to keep you slim – is one that is low (30% or less) in fat and particularly saturated fat, high (around 55%) in carbohydrate, preferably complex carbohydrates, and containing enough protein – up to 15%.

You can see at a glance what the proportions of these nutrients are in any food, e.g., you will see that Cheddar cheese contains nearly 75% fat and virtually no carbohydrate, so you will limit that food.

All foods listed which are high in saturated fat are preceded by an asterisk.

Remember also that not all foods high in carbohydrate are ideal – cakes, biscuits, desserts, sweets, for instance, may contain a high proportion of carbohydrate but this is usually simple carbohydrate, not complex, i.e., these foods are high in added · sugar, which isn't the kind of carbohydrate you want.

Remember that to keep hunger pangs at bay you need meals and snacks containing plenty of the low GI foods (refer back to page 43 for more information on this). Foods with a low GI are followed by a > symbol.

	% fat	% Carbohydrates	% Protein	Calories per stated portion	Grams of fat per stated portion
BISCUITS & BARS					
All per biscuit or bar					
* Digestive, large	40.0	52.0	8.0	75.0	3.3
* Digestive, chocolate, small	44.0	50.5	5.5	85.0	4.1
* Gingernut	30.0	65.0	5.0	45.0	1.5
* Harvest Crunch Bar	38.0	n/k	n/k	78.0	3.3
* Rich Tea	38.5	56.0	5.5	35.0	1.5
* Shortcake (oblong)	46.5	48.5	5.0	75.0	3.8
BREADS & CRISPBREADS					
All per 25g (1oz) unless otherwise stated					
Brown	9.0	75.0	16.0	56.0	0.55
French, white	1.2	83.3	15.5	62.5	trace
Granary	7.5	79.5	13.0	60.0	0.5
Malt loaf	12.0	74.5	13.5	62.0	0.82
Pitta, white, one	4.0	82.5	13.5	175.0	0.8
Pitta, brown, one	7.0	72.0	21.0	160.0	0.5
Wheatgerm (e.g. Hovis)	8.5	74.5	17.0	57.0	0.55
White	6.5	80.0	13.5	58.0	0.5
Wholemeal	11.0	73.0	16.0	54.0	0.67
Wholemeal, per slice from a large, medium-cut loaf	11.0	73.0	16.0	75.0	0.9
Wholemeal bap, one	11.0	73.0	16.0	120.0	1.5
Rice cake, one	7.0	85.5	7.5	24.0	0.2
Ryvita, one	11.5	77.5	11.0	25.0	0.2
* Cream cracker, one	33.0	58.0	9.0	40.0	1.5
* Oatcake, one	37.0	53.5	9.5	45.0	1.8
BREAKFAST CEREALS					
All per 25g (1oz) unless otherwise stated					
All-Bran	18.5	59.0	22.5	68.0	1.5
Branflakes	5.5	76.0	12.5	80.0	0.5
Cornflakes	4.0	86.5	9.5	92.0	0.4
Fruit 'n' Fibre	12.0	78.0	10.0	90.0	1.25

* High saturated fat

	% fat	% Carbohydrates	% Protein	Calories per stated portion	Grams of fat per stated portion
Muesli (no added sugar)	19.0	71.0	10.0	82.0	1.7
Porridge oats, raw	22.0	63.5	14.5	94.0	2.25
Porridge, made up with water, per 100ml (3½ fl oz)	18.0	70.0	12.0	44.0	0.9
Puffed Wheat	3.5	79.0	17.5	81.0	0.3
Shredded Wheat, one	8.5	78.5	13.0	80.0	0.75
Special K	6.0	75.5	18.5	97.0	0.6
Weetabix, one	9.0	77.5	13.5	65.0	0.65

CAKES & BAKERY ITEMS
All per item or slice

	% fat	% Carbohydrates	% Protein	Calories per stated portion	Grams of fat per stated portion
* Chocolate, rich, 50g (2oz) slice	53.0	42.0	5.0	c.230	13.6
* Croissant, 65g (2½ oz)	54.0	38.5	7.5	280.0	16.5
* Crumpet	3.5	83.0	13.5	100.0	0.5
* Doughnut, jam	41.0	52.5	6.5	c.260	12.0
* Eclair, chocolate	57.5	38.0	4.5	c.190	12.0
* Fruit cake, rich, 50g (2oz) slice	30.0	66.0	4.0	c.165	5.5
* Scone, plain	35.5	56.5	8.0	c.200	8.0
* Victoria sponge, 50g (2oz) slice	51.5	43.0	5.5	c.230	13.25

CHEESE
All per 25g (1oz) unless otherwise stated

	% fat	% Carbohydrates	% Protein	Calories per stated portion	Grams of fat per stated portion
* Brie or Camembert	69.5	trace	30.5	75.0	5.8
* Cheddar	74.5	trace	25.5	101.0	8.3
* Cheddar-style, half fat	50.5	trace	49.5	62.0	3.5
* Cheese spread	73.0	1.0	26.0	71.0	5.7
* Cottage cheese, standard	37.5	5.5	57.0	24.0	1.0
Cottage cheese, diet	18.0	trace	82.0	20.0	0.4
* Cream cheese, full-fat	97.0	trace	3.0	110.0	12.0
* Danish blue	74.0	trace	26.0	89.0	7.3
* Edam	68.0	trace	32.0	76.0	5.7
* Mozzarella, Italian	68.0	3.0	29.0	62.0	4.75
* Soft cheese, low-fat (e.g. Shape)	57.0	7.5	35.5	33.0	2.1
* Stilton	78.0	trace	22.0	115.0	10.0

* High saturated fat

		% fat	% Carbohydrates	% Protein	Calories per stated portion	Grams of fat per stated portion

DRESSINGS, SAUCES & PICKLES
All per tablespoon (20ml) unless otherwise stated

		% fat	% Carbohydrates	% Protein	Calories per stated portion	Grams of fat per stated portion
	Brown sauce	trace	95.5	4.5	20.0	trace
	Burger relish	trace	98.0	2.0	21.0	trace
	French dressing	100	trace	trace	130.0	14.5
*	Mayonnaise	99.0	trace	1.0	143.0	15.75
*	Mayonnaise, reduced-calorie	89.0	10.0	1.0	57.0	5.5
	Mayonnaise-style (Kraft)	28.0	66.0	6.0	15.0	0.5
	Salad cream	79.0	18.0	3.0	62.0	5.5
	Salad cream, reduced-calorie	66.5	31.0	2.5	26.0	2.0
	Soya sauce	6.0	71.0	23.0	11.0	trace
	Sweet pickle	2.0	96.0	2.0	26.0	trace
	Tartare sauce	83.0	14.0	3.0	47.0	4.4
	Tomato ketchup	1.0	91.0	8.0	20.0	trace
	White sauce	61.0	27.0	12.0	30.0	2.0

DRINKS
Alcoholic drinks

	% fat	% Carbohydrates	% Protein	Calories per stated portion	Grams of fat per stated portion
Beer, 275ml (1/2 pint)	trace	96.5	3.5	90.0	trace
Lager, 275ml (1/2 pint)	trace	97.5	2.5	90.0	trace
Spirits, all 1 measure	0.0	100.0	0.0	50.0	0.0
Stout, 275ml (1/2 pint)	trace	100.0	trace	90.0	trace
Wine, white, dry, average glass, 140ml (1/4 pint)	0.0	100.0	0.0	90.0	0.0
Wine, white, medium, average glass, 140ml (1/4 pint)	0.0	100.0	0.0	100.0	0.0
Wine, white, sweet, average glass, 140ml (1/4 pint)	0.0	99.0	1.01	40.0	0.0
Wine, red, average glass, 140ml (1/4 pint)	0.0	99.0	1.0	100.0	0.0
Port, 25ml (1fl oz)	0.0	100.0	trace	40.0	0.0
Sherry, 25ml (1fl oz)	0.0	100.0	trace	30.0	0.0

* High saturated fat

	% fat	% Carbohydrates	% Protein	Calories per stated portion	Grams of fat per stated portion
Beverages					
Tea	0.0	trace	trace	trace	0.0
Coffee, 1 teaspoon (5g)	0.0	41.0	59.0	2.5	0.0
* Hot chocolate, 200ml (7fl oz)	10.0	69.0	12.0	112.0	2.4
Low calorie instant hot chocolate,					
per sachet	24.0	56.0	20.0	40.0	1.0
Soft Drinks					
Cola, 1 can (330ml)	0.0	100.0	0.0	135.0	0.0
Lemonade, 1 glass (200ml)	0.0	100.0	0.0	50.0	0.0
Orange squash, 1 glass (200ml)	0.0	100.0	0.0	60.0	0.0
Fruit Juices					
All per average glass (125ml)					
Apple	0.0	97.0	3.0	50.0	0.0
Grape	0.0	97.0	3.0	75.0	0.0
Grapefruit	0.0	96.0	4.0	50.0	0.0
Mixed citrus	0.0	96.0	4.0	50.0	0.0
Mixed vegetable	0.0	85.0	15.0	25.0	0.0
Orange >	0.0	95.0	5.0	50.0	0.0
Pineapple	0.0	97.0	3.0	55.0	0.0
Tomato	0.0	83.0	17.0	25.0	0.0
EGGS					
All per egg					
* Size 2	67.0	trace	33.0	90.0	6.8
* Size 3	67.0	trace	33.0	80.0	6.0
* Size 4	67.0	trace	33.0	75.0	5.5
* Size 3, fried, drained	78.0	trace	22.0	120.0	10.5
* Size 3, scrambled with 7g (1/4 oz)					
low-fat spread and 25ml (1fl oz)					
skimmed milk	64.0	4.0	32.0	115.0	9.0

* High saturated fat   > low GI

	% fat	% Carbohydrates	% Protein	Calories per stated portion	Grams of fat per stated portion
FATS & OILS					
All per 25g (1oz) unless otherwise stated					
* Butter	100.0	trace	trace	185.0	20.5
Low-fat spread	100.0	0.0	0.0	91.0	10.0
Very low-fat spread	100.0	0.0	0.0	57.0	6.3
* Margarine, hard	100.0	trace	trace	132.0	20.25
Margarine, sunflower or					
olive oil type	100.0	trace	trace	182.0	20.25
Oils, all kinds	100.0	0.0	trace	225.0	25.0
FISH & SEAFOOD					
All per 100g (3¹/₂ oz) unless otherwise stated					
Cod, coley, haddock or					
monkfish fillet	8.0	0.0	92.0	76.0	0.7
Deep-fried fish in batter	47.0	14.0	39.0	200.0	10.3
Fish finger, grilled, one	38.0	34.0	28.0	50.0	2.0
Fish, frozen, in light batter,					
baked or grilled, one portion	51.5	28.5	20.0	203.0	11.6
Haddock, smoked fillet	8.0	0.0	92.0	100.0	0.9
Herring, fillet	71.0	0.0	29.0	234.0	18.5
Kipper, grilled fillet	50.0	0.0	50.0	205.0	11.4
Pilchards in tomato sauce	38.5	2.0	59.5	126.0	5.4
Plaice fillet	18.0	0.0	82.0	93.0	1.9
Salmon, fresh, fillet	59.0	0.0	41.0	197.0	13.0
Salmon, smoked	28.5	0.0	71.5	142.0	4.5
Salmon, pink, canned	47.5	0.0	52.5	155.0	8.2
Scampi, deep-fried	50.0	34.0	16.0	316.0	17.6
Trout, one average (225g, 8oz)	30.0	0.0	70.0	200.0	6.75
Tuna in brine, drained	3.0	0.0	97.0	114.0	0.35
Tuna in oil, drained	47.0	0.0	53.0	210.0	11.0
Whitebait, deep-fried	81.0	4.0	15.0	525.0	47.5

* High saturated fat

	% fat	% Carbohydrates	% Protein	Calories per stated portion	Grams of fat per stated portion
Seafood					
Crabmeat, canned	10.0	0.0	90.0	81.0	0.9
Crabmeat, fresh	37.0	0.0	63.0	127.0	5.2
Prawns, shelled	15.0	0.0	85.0	107.0	1.8
Mussels, shelled	20.5	trace	79.5	87.0	2.0
Scallops, shelled	12.0	trace	89.0	105.0	1.4
Squid	15.0	trace	85.0	82.0	1.4
FRUIT					
All per item unless otherwise stated					
Apple, dessert >	trace	97.0	3.0	45.0	trace
Apple, cooking, 25g (1oz)	trace	97.0	3.0	40.0	trace
Apricot, fresh >	trace	93.0	7.0	10.0	trace
Apricots, dried, 25g (1oz)	trace	89.5	10.5	45.0	trace
Banana, small	3.5	91.0	5.5	60.0	0.2
Banana, medium	3.5	91.0	5.5	80.0	0.3
Banana, large	3.5	91.0	5.5	100.0	0.4
Blackberries, 25g (1oz)	trace	83.01	7.0	7.0	trace
Blackcurrants, 25g (1oz)	trace	88.0	12.0	7.0	trace
Currants, dried, 25g (1oz)	trace	97.0	3.0	60.0	trace
Cherries, 25g (1oz) >	trace	95.0	5.0	10.0	trace
Damsons, 25g (1oz)	trace	95.0	5.0	8.0	trace
Dates, stoned, 25g (1oz)	trace	96.5	3.5	62.0	trace
Dates, each, fresh or dry	trace	96.5	3.5	15.0	trace
Fig, fresh	trace	87.0	13.0	10.0	trace
Fig, dry	trace	93.0	7.0	53.0	trace
Gooseberries, dessert, 25g (1oz)	trace	75.0	25.0	4.0	trace
Gooseberries, cooking, 25g (1oz)	trace	93.0	7.0	9.0	trace
Grapefruit, half >	trace	90.0	10.0	20.0	trace
Grapes, 25g (1oz)	trace	96.0	4.0	16.0	trace
Kiwi fruit	6.0	86.0	8.0	25.0	trace
Lemon	trace	80.0	20.0	15.0	trace

> low GI

	% fat	% Carbohydrates	% Protein	Calories per stated portion	Grams of fat per stated portion
Lime	trace	80.0	20.0	10.0	trace
Mango	trace	97.0	3.0	100.0	trace
Melon, 200g (7oz), slice	trace	90.0	10.0	25.0	trace
Nectarine	trace	93.0	7.0	50.0	trace
Orange >	trace	92.0	8.0	50.0	trace
Peach >	trace	92.0	8.0	50.0	trace
Pear, medium	trace	98.0	2.0	50.0	trace
Pineapple, one ring	trace	95.0	5.0	25.0	trace
Plum, one dessert >	trace	94.0	6.0	20.0	trace
Prunes, stoned, 25g (1oz)	trace	94.0	6.0	40.0	trace
Prune, each	trace	94.0	6.0	10.0	trace
Raisins, 25g (1oz)	trace	98.0	2.0	61.0	trace
Raspberries, 25g (1oz)	trace	84.0	16.0	6.0	trace
Rhubarb, 1 large stick (100g, 3 1/2 oz)	trace	62.5	37.5	6.0	trace
Satsuma or tangerine	trace	91.0	9.0	20.0	trace
Strawberries, 25g (1oz)	trace	90.0	10.0	6.0	trace
Sultanas, 25g (1oz)	trace	97.0	3.0	62.0	trace

GRAINS

All per 25g (1oz) unless otherwise stated

	% fat	% Carbohydrates	% Protein	Calories per stated portion	Grams of fat per stated portion
Bulgar, couscous, dry weight >	4.5	83.0	12.5	88.0	0.4
Buckwheat >	4	87.0	9	91.0	0.4
Barley, pot >	2.5	86.5	11	87.0	0.25
Flour, white	3.0	86.0	11.0	87.0	0.3
Flour, wholemeal	6.0	77.5	16.5	80.0	0.5
Pasta, all shapes, white, dry weight	3.0	83.0	14.0	95.0	0.25
Pasta, white, boiled	3.0	83.0	14.0	29.0	trace
Pasta, all shapes, brown, dry weight	6.0	n/k	n/k	85.0	0.6
Pasta, brown, boiled	8.5	72.5	18.0	32.0	0.3
Pearl barley, dry weight	4.0	87.0	9.0	90.0	0.4

> low GI

	% fat	% Carbohydrates	% Protein	Calories per stated portion	Grams of fat per stated portion
Rice, white, dry weight	2.5	90.0	7.5	90.0	0.25
Rice, white, boiled	2.0	90.0	8.0	30.0	trace
Rice, brown, dry weight	7.0	85.0	6.0	90.0	0.7
Rice, brown, boiled	7.0	86.0	7.0	30.0	0.45
Rice salad from deli	13.0	75.0	12.0	35.0	0.5
Spaghetti in tomato sauce, 215g (7¹/2 oz) can	10.5	77.5	12.0	127.0	1.5

MEAT & POULTRY

All per 25g (1oz) unless otherwise stated

	% fat	% Carbohydrates	% Protein	Calories per stated portion	Grams of fat per stated portion
* Beef, minced, average	60.0	0.0	40.0	57.0	3.8
* Beef, minced, extra lean	35.0	0.0	65.0	47.0	1.8
Beef, roast, lean only	25.0	0.0	75.0	40.0	1.1
* Beef steak, grilled, lean only	32.0	0.0	68.0	42.0	1.5
* Beefburger, grilled, one frozen, 50g (2oz)	64.0	5.0	31.0	120.0	8.5
* Bacon, back, trimmed, grilled	58.0	0.0	42.0	73.0	4.7
* Bacon, streaky, grilled	77.0	0.0	23.0	105.0	9.0
Chicken fillet, no skin, raw	30.0	0.0	70.0	30.0	1.0
Chicken, grilled, average breast portion (no wing), 200g (7oz)					
with skin	60.0	0.0	40.0	225.0	15.0
without skin	42.0	0.0	58.0	150.0	7.0
Chicken, roast, meat only	33.0	0.0	67.0	37.0	1.3
* Corned beef	50.0	0.0	50.0	54.0	3.0
Duck, breast fillet	46.0	0.0	54.0	47.0	2.4
Duck, roast, meat and skin	77.0	0.0	23.0	85.0	7.2
Gammon steak, grilled, lean only	27.0	0.0	73.0	43.0	1.3
* Ham, extra lean	37.5	0.0	62.5	30.0	1.25
Kidneys, lamb's	27.0	0.0	73.0	22.0	0.67
* Lamb, one average trimmed chop	50.0	0.0	50.0	120.0	6.8
* Lamb, leg roast, lean only	38.0	0.0	62.0	48.0	2.0
* Lamb, shoulder, roast	75.0	0.0	25.0	80.0	6.5

* High saturated fat

	% fat	% Carbohydrates	% Protein	Calories per stated portion	Grams of fat per stated portion
Liver, lamb's	52.0	3.0	45.0	45.0	2.5
* Liver sausage	78.0	5.5	16.5	77.0	6.7
* Luncheon meat	77.5	6.5	16.0	78.0	6.7
* Pork, roast, lean only	34.0	0.0	66.0	46.0	1.7
* Pork fillet, raw	43.0	0.0	57.0	37.0	1.75
Rabbit (excluding bone)	29.0	0.0	71.0	31.0	1.0
Salami	83.0	1.0	16.0	122.0	11.3
Sausages, low-fat, grilled, per chipolata	43.0	23.0	34.0	50.0	2.4
Sausages, pork, grilled, per chipolata	70.0	13.5	16.5	75.0	5.8
Sausages, beef, grilled per chipolata	59.0	21.5	19.5	70.0	4.5
Turkey, light meat (no skin)	9.5	0.0	90.5	26.0	0.27
Turkey, dark meat (no skin)	28.0	0.0	72.0	28.0	0.9
* Tongue	70.0	0.0	30.0	53.0	4.0
Veal fillet, raw	22.0	0.0	78.0	27.0	0.6
Venison fillet	29.0	0.0	71.0	49.0	1.6

MILK & CREAM
All per 25g (1fl oz) unless otherwise stated

	% fat	% Carbohydrates	% Protein	Calories per stated portion	Grams of fat per stated portion
Milk, whole >	52.5	27.0	20.5	16.0	1.0
Milk, semi-skimmed >	31.5	39.0	29.5	11.5	0.4
Milk, skimmed >	2.0	57.0	41.0	8.0	trace
Soya milk >	45.0	n/k	n/k	14.0	0.7
Instant low-fat milk, dry, per tablespoon	3.0	56.0	41.0	18.0	trace
* Single cream	90.0	5.5	4.5	53.0	5.3
* Double cream	97.0	1.5	1.5	112.0	12.0
* Aerosol cream	87.0	10.0	3.0	16.0	1.5
* Sour cream	88.0	7.0	5.0	51.0	5.0
* Crème fraîche, low-fat	79.0	n/k	n/k	42.5	3.75

* High saturated fat   > low GI

	% fat	% Carbohydrates	% Protein	Calories per stated portion	Grams of fat per stated portion
NUTS & CRISPS					
All per 25g (1oz). Nuts all shelled weight					
Almonds	85.0	3.0	12.0	141.0	13.3
Brazils	89.5	2.5	8.0	155.0	15.3
Chestnuts	14.0	81.0	5.0	42.0	0.67
Hazelnuts	85.0	7.0	8.0	95.0	9.0
Peanuts, fresh or roasted	77.5	5.5	17.0	142.0	12.2
Walnuts	89.0	3.0	8.0	131.0	9.0
Crisps, standard	60.5	34.5	5.0	133.0	9.0
Low fat crisps	56.0	36.5	7.5	105.0	6.5
PASTRY & PIZZA					
* Flaky, 25g (1oz)	64.5	31.5	4.0	106.0	7.6
* Shortcrust, 25g (1oz)	55.0	40.0	5.0	113.0	7.0
Filo, 25g (1oz)	9.5	78.0	12.5	67.0	0.7
* Cornish pasty, one small, 130g (5oz)	55.5	35.0	9.5	430.0	26.5
* Jam tart, one	35.0	61.0	4.0	150.0	5.8
* Mince pie, one	43.0	53.0	4.0	200.0	9.5
* Pizza, cheese & tomato 100g (3½ oz) slice	44.0	40.0	16.0	235.0	11.5
* Pork pie, one individual, 140g (5oz)	64.5	25.0	10.5	530.0	37.8
* Quiche, 100g (3½ oz) slice	65.0	20.0	15.0	390.0	28.0
* Sausage roll, one large	68.0	26.0	6.0	270.0	20.5
* Steak & kidney one individual pie, 130g (5oz)	59.0	30.0	11.0	480.0	31.5
PUDDING & DESSERTS					
* Black Forest Gâteau, 100g (3½ oz)	53.0	42.0	5.0	310.0	18.2
* Cheesecake, 50g (2oz)	75.0	21.0	4.0	210.0	17.5

* High saturated fat

	% fat	% Carbohydrates	% Protein	Calories per stated portion	Grams of fat per stated portion
Custard, bought, 100ml	34.0	53.0	13.0	120.0	4.5
* Fruit pie, 100g (3½ oz)	38.0	57.5	4.5	180.0	7.6
* Ice cream, vanilla, 50g (2oz)	35.5	55.5	9.0	83.0	3.3
* Trifle, 100g (3½ oz)	34.0	57.0	9.0	160.0	6.1

PULSES – BEANS, PEAS & LENTILS
All per 25g (1oz)

	% fat	% Carbohydrates	% Protein	Calories per stated portion	Grams of fat per stated portion
Baked beans in tomato sauce >	6.0	61.0	33.0	16.0	0.1
Butter beans, canned or boiled >	2.5	67.5	30.0	23.0	trace
Chick peas, canned or boiled >	18.0	60.0	22.0	40.0	0.8
Haricot beans, canned or boiled >	5.0	67.0	28.0	23.0	0.1
Kidney beans, canned or boiled >	4.5	59.5	36.0	25.0	0.1
Lentils, dry weight >	3.0	65.5	31.5	76.0	0.25
Lentils, boiled >	4.5	64.5	31.0	25.0	0.1
Split peas, boiled >	2.5	69.5	28.0	30.0	trace

SOUPS
All per 300g (11oz) serving

	% fat	% Carbohydrates	% Protein	Calories per stated portion	Grams of fat per stated portion
* Cream of chicken	59.0	29.0	12.0	175.0	11.5
* Cream of tomato	45.0	46.0	9.0	173.0	8.7
Lentil >	2.5	72.5	25.0	115.0	0.3
Minestrone	29.5	55.0	15.5	90.0	2.9
Vegetable	14.5	72.5	13.0	110.0	1.8

SPREADS
All per 25g (1oz) unless otherwise stated

	% fat	% Carbohydrates	% Protein	Calories per stated portion	Grams of fat per stated portion
Jam	0.0	99.0	1.0	65.0	0.0
* Liver pâté	67.5	1.5	31.0	80.0	6.0
Marmalade	0.0	100.0	trace	65.0	0.0
Marmite, 1 teaspoon (5g)	3.5	4.0	92.5	9.0	trace
Peanut butter	77.5	8.0	14.5	156.0	13.4
Taramasalata	94.0	3.5	2.5	110.0	11.5

* High saturated fat   > low GI

	% fat	% Carbohydrates	% Protein	Calories per stated portion	Grams of fat per stated portion
SUGARS & CONFECTIONERY					
All per 25g (1oz) unless otherwise stated					
* Chocolate, milk or plain	51.5	42.0	6.5	132.0	7.5
Honey	0.0	99.5	0.5	72.0	0.0
Sugar	0.0	100.0	0.0	98.0	0.0
Sugar, per teaspoon	0.0	100.0	0.0	20.0	0.0
Sweets, boiled	0.0	100.0	0.0	82.0	0.0
Syrup	0.0	100.0	0.0	75.0	0.0
Toffee	36.0	62.0	2.0	107.0	4.3
VEGETABLES					
All per 25g (1oz) unless otherwise stated					
Artichoke, globe, one whole					
(edible parts)	1.0	70.0	29.0	15.0	trace
Artichoke, Jerusalem	trace	64.5	35.5	4.5	trace
Asparagus, one spear, 50g (2oz)	trace	24.0	75.5	4.5	trace
Aubergine	trace	80.0	20.0	3.5	trace
Avocado, half medium,					
65g (2¹/₂ oz) >	89.0	3.0	8.0	145.0	14.4
Beans, broad >	10.5	55.5	34.0	12.0	0.1
Beans, French >	trace	59.0	41.0	10.0	trace
Beans, runner >	7.0	53.0	40.0	5.0	trace
Beansprouts	trace	29.0	71.0	7.0	trace
Beetroot	trace	84.0	16.0	11.0	trace
Broccoli >	trace	31.0	69.0	4.5	trace
Brussels sprouts >	trace	36.0	62.0	4.5	trace
Cabbage, white >	trace	65.0	35.0	5.0	trace
Cabbage, dark >	trace	50.0	50.0	6.0	trace
Cabbage, red >	trace	66.0	34.0	5.0	trace
Carrots	trace	88.0	12.0	6.0	trace
Cauliflower >	trace	42.0	58.0	3.0	trace
Celery	trace	61.0	39.0	2.0	trace
Chicory	trace	62.0	38.0	2.0	trace

* High saturated fat   > low GI

	% fat	% Carbohydrates	% Protein	Calories per stated portion	Grams of fat per stated portion
Chinese leaves	trace	50.0	50.0	3.0	trace
Corn on the cob, one	17.0	70.0	13.0	80.0	1.5
Courgettes >	3.5	67.5	29.0	5.0	0.1
Cucumber	9.0	67.0	24.0	2.0	trace
Leek >	trace	72.0	28.0	8.0	trace
Lettuce	30.0	37.5	32.5	3.0	0.1
Marrow	trace	87.0	13.0	4.0	trace
Mushrooms >	41.5	n/k	55.0	3.0	0.1
Mustard and cress, whole box	trace	34.0	64.0	5.0	trace
Onion >	trace	85.0	15.0	6.0	trace
Onion, spring, one	trace	91.0	9.0	3.0	trace
Parsnip	trace	86.5	13.5	12.0	trace
Peas, shelled, fresh or frozen >	7.0	55.0	38.0	13.0	0.1
Pepper, green >	22.5	53.5	24.0	4.0	0.1
Pepper, other colours >	11.0	77.0	12.0	8.0	0.1
Potatoes					
boiled	1.0	92.0	7.0	20.0	trace
mashed	38.0	57.0	5.0	30.0	1.25
instant mashed (made-up)	9.5	79.0	11.5	16.0	0.2
baked, average 225g (8oz)	1.0	89.5	9.5	190.0	0.2
roast, one chunk	27.5	65.0	7.5	80.0	2.4
chips, average cut, cooked in oil,					
25g (1oz)	41.5	55.0	3.5	65.0	3.0
chips, oven	32.0	62.5	5.5	49.0	1.75
Radish	trace	70.0	30.0	4.0	trace
Spinach >	14.5	17.5	68.0	7.0	0.1
Swede	trace	77.0	13.0	5.0	trace
Sweet potato	6.5	88.5	5.0	21.0	0.15
Sweetcorn kernels	15.0	69.5	15.5	30.0	0.5
Tomato, one average	trace	75.0	25.0	7.0	trace
Tomatoes, canned	1.0	62.5	36.5	3.0	trace
Turnip	22.0	62.0	16.0	4.0	trace
Watercress	trace	17.0	83.0	3.0	trace

> low GI

	% fat	% Carbohydrates	% Protein	Calories per stated portion	Grams of fat per stated portion
VEGETARIAN PRODUCTS					
Nut loaf, 100g (3½ oz)	41.0	41.0	18.0	210.0	9.5
Quorn, 25g (1oz)	34.0	8.0	58.0	21.0	0.8
Sosmix, made up, 100g (3½ oz)	59.0	24.0	17.0	170.0	11.2
Tofu, 25g (1oz) >	53.0	3.0	44.0	17.0	1.0
TVP mince, reconstituted 25g (1oz) >	2.5	39.0	58.5	17.0	trace
VegeBurger, average 50g (2oz)	45.0	22.5	32.5	81.0	4.0
YOGURT & FROMAGE FRAIS					
All per 25g (1oz) unless otherwise stated					
Fromage frais, diet fruit, 100g tub	2.0	39.5	58.5	43.0	trace
Fromage frais, natural, 8% fat >	64.0	9.0	27.0	28.0	2.0
Fromage frais, natural, very low fat	4.0	22.0	74.0	12.0	trace
Yogurt, diet fruit, 125g tub	2.0	54.0	44.0	51.0	trace
Yogurt, low fat, natural >	13.5	48.0	38.5	13.0	trace
Yogurt, whole milk, natural >	52.0	25.0	23.0	17.0	1.0
Yogurt, strained Greek	61.0			33.0	2.5

> low GI

CASE HISTORIES

Case History One

Jenny Simmons, forty-four, works in the travel industry and has a teenage son. Before *Bodysense*, Jenny said, 'I'm not vastly overweight but I am suffering from that old problem of "middle aged spread" on my thighs and tummy, so I can no longer get into most of my size 12 wardrobe. I'm also unfit; I belong to a gym but rarely go. I'd love to get fit, shape up and get back into my clothes without losing much weight from my top half.'

In 12 weeks, Jenny did exactly that although suffering from a long bout of 'flu midway through the programme. Following the *Bodysense* guidelines on going WITH her body rather than fighting it, Jenny began to enjoy exercising and soon managed to control her least-healthy eating habits, such as eating biscuits and cakes at her desk. 'Not that I've been starving or going without the odd treat. I eat something when I need it now. And the exercise has paid off – I've just had my first-ever skiing holiday and could walk up mountains without puffing and blowing and had no aching limbs.

Jenny's hips and thighs are noticeably firmer and smaller. 'I'm happy with my shape now; I don't want to lose any more weight. I've enjoyed the *Bodysense* programme – it was just what I needed.'

Case History Two

District nurse **Jane Lucy** is thirty-three years old and has two pre-school children. Before she tried *Bodysense*, she said, 'I find it very hard to diet with my busy life and though I intend to exercise it never lasts. Please help – I'm desperate not to be a "fat mum" for ever.'

Three months later, despite being sterilised early in the programme which meant no exercise for a while, and despite personal problems, Jane had managed to lose a stone (7 kg) plus eleven inches off her statistics.

'I loved the *Bodysense* programme,' she said. 'It suits my moods and is ideal for helping me to avoid the main pitfalls of normal dieting – hunger and guilt. I loved being able to eat when I wanted to; that was the biggest bonus, but because the food was healthier I could still lose weight. I've even enjoyed the exercise – through the winter I used my exercise bike and did skipping. I thoroughly enjoyed the whole thing and would recommend it to anyone,'

CASE HISTORY ONE: Jenny Simmons from Hounslow, Middlesex

Before **Weight:** 68kg (10 stone 2$^{1}/_{2}$lbs) **Statistics:** 34–28–38

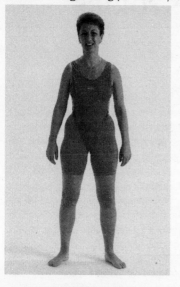
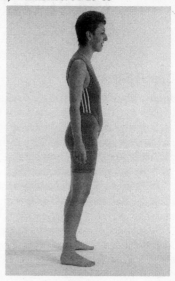

After 3 Months **Weight:** 61kg (9 stone 9$^{1}/_{2}$ lbs) **Statistics:** 34–27$^{1}/_{2}$–37

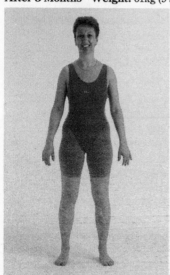
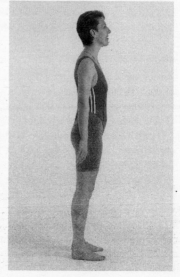

'Now at last I am in control of my eating.'

CASE HISTORY TWO: Jane Lucy from Wrexham, Clwyd
Before **Weight:** 67kg (10 stone 7lbs) **Statistics:** 40–35–40

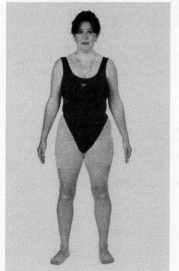
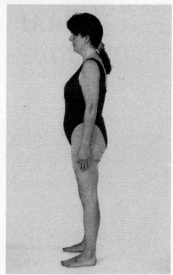

After 3 Months **Weight:** 60kg (9 stone 7lbs) **Statistics:** 36–30–38

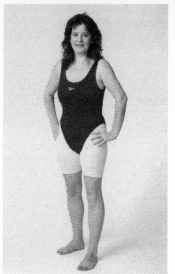
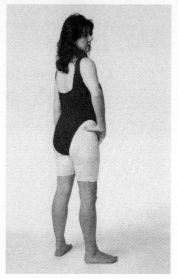

'This is the ideal programme for any woman.'

PRAISE FOR
THE BODYSENSE DIET

'A great, new, down-to-earth guide that addresses all the problems women face when trying to lose weight.'
Caroline Hogg, Beauty Editor, **woman** *Magazine.*

'*Bodysense* makes absolute sense to me; *Slimmer* readers often say their best efforts at dieting are defeated by unpredictable appetite ups and downs. Judith Wills explains all.'
Claire Crowther, Editor, Slimmer *Magazine.*

'Commonsense for today's woman.'
The Express.

INDEX

Page numbers in *italic* refer to the illustrations